Basic Endocrinology

Other books of interest

Pharmaceutical Biotechnology – An Introduction for Pharmacists and Pharmaceutical Scientists
D.J.A. Crommelin and R.D. Sindelar

Immunology – for Pharmacy Students
W.C. Shen and S. Louie

Forthcoming

Drug Delivery and Targeting – for Pharmacists and Pharmaceutical Scientists
A.M. Hillery, A.W. Lloyd and J. Swarbrick

Basic Endocrinology
for Students of Pharmacy and Allied Health Sciences

Andrew Constanti *(The School of Pharmacy, University of London, London, UK)*

and

Andrzej Bartke *(Department of Physiology, Southern Illinois University, School of Medicine, Carbondale, IL, USA)*

with clinical contributions and case studies by

Romesh Khardori *(Division of Endocrinology, Department of Internal Medicine, Southern Illinois University, School of Medicine, Springfield, IL, USA)*

ho
ap **harwood academic publishers**
Australia • Canada • China • France • Germany • India • Japan • Luxembourg • Malaysia
The Netherlands • Russia • Singapore • Switzerland • Thailand

Amsteldijk 166
1st Floor
1079 LH Amsterdam
The Netherlands

British Library Cataloguing in Publication Data

A catalogue record for this book is available from the British Library.

ISBN: 90-5702-251-6 (softcover)

To Heather, Lisa and Sophia

Table of Contents

Preface   *xv*

Chapter 1:   **Introduction and General Principles**   *1*

The Mode of Action of Hormones on Cells   *1*
Control of Hormone Secretion: The Concept of Feedback
   Mechanisms   *3*
   Direct Negative Feedback   *3*
   Indirect Negative Feedback   *4*
   Positive Feedback   *5*
Review Questions   *6*
References   *6*

Chapter 2:   **The Hypothalamus and Pituitary**   *7*

Structure and Histology   *7*
   Histology   *8*
The Hypothalamic-Hypophyseal Portal System   *8*
Hypothalamic Releasing and Inhibiting Hormones that
   Influence the Anterior Pituitary   *8*
   Gonadotrophin Releasing Hormone   *8*
   Corticotrophin Releasing Hormone   *9*
   Thyrotrophin Releasing Hormone   *9*
   Prolactin-Releasing/Inhibiting Factors   *9*
   Growth Hormone Releasing Hormone   *9*
Hormones of the Anterior Pituitary   *10*
   Gonadotrophins   *10*
   Thyrotrophin (Thyroid Stimulating Hormone, TSH)   *10*
   Corticotrophin (Adrenocorticotrophic Hormone, ACTH)   *11*
   Prolactin   *13*
   Growth Hormone   *14*
Hormones of the Posterior Pituitary   *16*
   Vasopressin   *16*
   Oxytocin   *17*
Review Questions   *18*
Clinical Case Studies   *18*
References   *23*

Chapter 3:   **The Adrenal Gland**   *25*

Structure and Histology   *25*
   Histology   *25*
Biosynthesis and Release of Adrenocortical Hormones   *26*
   Control of Release   *26*

Glucocorticoids *26*
   Carbohydrate Metabolism *26*
   Protein Metabolism *28*
   Fat (Lipid) Metabolism *28*
   Anti-inflammatory and Immunosuppressive Actions *28*
   Response to Stress *30*
   Mechanism of Action *30*
   Clinical Disorders *30*
Mineralocorticoids *33*
   Mechanism of Action *34*
   Clinical Disorders *36*
Review Questions *37*
Clinical Case Studies *37*
References *43*

Chapter 4: **The Thyroid Gland** *45*

Structure and Histology *45*
   Histology *45*
Biosynthesis and Release of Thyroid Hormones *45*
   Control of Release *47*
Thyroid Hormones *47*
   Calorigenesis *47*
   Influence on Metabolism *47*
   Maturation of the Central Nervous System (CNS) *48*
   Skeletal Growth and Maturation *48*
   Mechanism of Action of Thyroid Hormones *48*
   Clinical Disorders *49*
      Thyroid Hyposecretion *49*
      Thyroid Hypersecretion *50*
      'Sick Euthyroid' Syndrome *52*
Review Questions *53*
Clinical Case Studies *53*
References *57*

Chapter 5: **Endocrine Secretions of the Pancreas** *59*

Structure and Histology *59*
   Histology *59*
Pancreatic Hormones *59*
   Insulin *59*
   Glucagon *64*
   Other Islet β-cell Peptides *65*
Clinical Disorders *67*
   Glucagon Hyposecretion *67*
   Insulin Deficiency *67*
   Secondary Diabetes *68*
   Primary Diabetes Mellitus *68*
   Gestational Diabetes *69*
   Some Late Clinical Features of Diabetes *69*
   Insulin Excess *70*
   Diagnosis and Monitoring of Diabetes *70*

Treatment of Diabetes   72
Acute Complications of Diabetic Therapy   75
Review Questions   77
Clinical Case Studies   78
References   83

Chapter 6:   **The Gonads and Reproduction**   85

The Male Reproductive System   85
Structure and Histology   85
Control of Spermatogenesis and Hormone Release   86
Androgens: Testosterone   87
Clinical Disorders   88
Some Clinical Uses of Androgens   88
The Female Reproductive System   90
Structure and Histology   90
The Ovarian Cycle and Hormone Release   90
The Uterine Cycle   90
Hormonal Regulation of Menstrual Cycle   91
Hormonal Changes during Pregnancy   92
The Menopause   93
Female Sex Hormones   94
Clinical Disorders   95
Some Clinical Uses of Oestrogens and Progestogens   96
Intrauterine Devices (IUDs)   101
Pregnancy Testing   103
Review Questions   104
Clinical Case Studies   105
References   109

Chapter 7:   **The Parathyroid Glands, Vitamin D and Hormonal Control of Calcium Metabolism**   111

The Parathyroid Glands   111
Structure and Histology   111
Parathyroid Hormone   111
Principal Actions   112
Bone Cells Affected by Parathyroid Hormone   113
Mechanism of Action   113
Clinical Disorders   114
Calcitonin   116
Principal Actions   116
Clinical Disorders   116
Therapeutic Uses   116
Vitamin D   117
Principal Actions   118
Clinical Disorders   118
Keratinocyte Differentiation   120
Other Hormones Affecting Calcium Homeostasis   121
Gonadal Steroids   121
Glucocorticoids   121
Growth Hormone   121

Osteoporosis   *121*
  Risk Factors   *122*
    Bone Density Measurements   *122*
    Prevention and Treatment   *122*
Review Questions   *124*
Clinical Case Studies   *125*
References   *129*

Abbreviations list   *131*
UK/USA spelling   *133*
Index   *135*

Preface

This textbook is primarily intended to provide undergraduate students of pharmacy with a clear and concise account of basic endocrine function and dysfunction, at a level sufficient to meet the requirements of first- or second year qualifying examinations. It is not intended to replace standard texts, but merely to serve as an accompaniment and convenient revision guide.

The text is based on a series of endocrinology lectures delivered to Pharmacy and Toxicology/pharmacology students at *The School of Pharmacy, University of London*, and is presented in an original stylised format to allow for easier reading/learning; this approach has received a highly favourable response from students and colleagues here over the past ten years, and was the main impetus for undertaking this new book endeavour.

Basic Endocrinology for Students of Pharmacy and Allied Health Sciences is arranged into seven chapters: the first provides a basic introduction to the organization of the endocrine system and the concept of feedback regulation of hormone release. Subsequent sections deal, in turn, with the hormone secretions of each major endocrine gland, covering the mechanisms that control hormone release, the principal actions of the hormones in the body, the most commonly recognised clinical disorders that can arise when hormones are under or oversecreted, and how these disorders may be diagnosed and managed therapeutically. Where effects of hormones or major signs/symptoms of endocrine diseases are described, the text is separated into distinct sections for easier identification.

This chosen format is especially intended to assist students in learning information in a logical ordered sequence. Review questions and clinical case studies (fictitious) dealing with common endocrine diseases (prepared with the consultation and kind collaboration of Dr. Romesh Khardori) are included at the end of every main chapter as a further aid to learning and revision. Drug names and doses (appropriate at the time of writing) of currently available pharmaceutical preparations with an endocrine basis, and those used to treat endocrine diseases, are also included throughout, based on current information provided in the *British National Formulary (BNF; September 1996)* and the *Monthly Index of Medical Specialities (MIMS; June 1997)*; [equivalent preparations used in the USA are listed for the convenience of overseas readers, based on the *Physicians Desk Reference, 1996*]. Since drug information may be subject to updates (with some preparations being modified or withdrawn), readers are recommended to check with more current editions of *MIMS, BNF* or *Desk Reference* for descriptions of currently available formulations and their usage.

Although the text presented has been based on information from recent articles, reviews and book chapters, it is not meant to provide a comprehensive coverage of the literature, and more advanced readers are advised to consult the original references quoted at the end of each chapter for further source of information.

The field of human endocrinology is a vast and rapidly expanding area, and to achieve our goal of brevity and a clear focus on key concepts (essential for examinations), it was necessary to sacrifice much detailed physiological and molecular detail on the synthesis, release, transport and mechanism of hormone action. We hope that the resultant simplified, logical presentation style we have adopted in dealing with the subject (not easily found in other endocrine texts) will make the learning of endocrinology a more interesting and pleasurable experience!

We would like to thank Mr. Derek King (Department of Pharmacology, The School of Pharmacy) for useful assistance and advice in the preparation of the original illustrations.

Andrew Constanti
London, UK

Andrzej Bartke
Carbondale, Illinois, USA
Romesh Khardori
Springfield, Illinois, USA

I Introduction and General Principles

Effective communication between different parts of the body is absolutely essential for the functioning of any multicellular organism. In vertebrates, including humans, this communication is maintained by nerve fibres and *hormones*; endocrinology is concerned with the nature of these hormones and with *hormonal communication*.

Hormones are specialized chemical substances that are produced by particular ductless internal glands of the body (or groups of secretory cells), and then discharged *directly* into the bloodstream (in response to a stimulus) by a process of endocrine secretion. They are then carried via the circulation to other parts of the body where, in extremely small quantities (10^{-7}–10^{-12} mol/l), they exert specific regulatory effects on their selected 'target' cells, which possess particular recognition features (*hormone receptors*). Some hormones however, act more generally in the body, rather than on a specific target tissue. By contrast, *exocrine* glands discharge their secretions via ducts, to the external surface of the body (e.g. milk, sweat) or into the intestinal lumen (e.g. digestive enzymes).

Modern research in endocrinology also includes studies of *locally-produced growth factors*, and other substances that are involved in communication between different cell types *within* an organ (so-called *paracrine* hormones); these substances would not therefore fit into the 'classical' concept of hormones and endocrine control.

The four principal physiological areas of hormonal function include the control of reproduction, the general growth and development of the body, the regulation of electrolyte composition of bodily fluids and the control of energy metabolism.

Chemically, hormones may be classified into three main groups: *amino acid (tyrosine) derivatives* (from the adrenal medulla and thyroid gland), *steroids*, structurally related to cholesterol (from the sex glands and the adrenal cortex) and *proteins/polypeptides* (from the pancreas and pituitary gland). Many polypeptide hormones are synthesized and stored by the endocrine cell as inactive longer chain 'pro-hormones', from which the hormone itself is eventually released by enzymatic cleavage.

As a means of communication between cells, the endocrine hormonal system may be contrasted with the nervous system, where cells communicate electrically by means of precisely defined nerve fibres, releasing specific neurotransmitters onto other effector cells that they innervate (e.g. nerve, muscle or gland cells). Nervous communication becomes important when a *fast*, rapidly modulated message is required e.g. that involved in skeletal muscle movement (operating within milliseconds), whereas hormonal communication would seem better suited for providing a more *slowly developing* (from seconds to several days), widespread, and longer-term regulatory action. There are also occasions where the two systems can be seen to interact: i.e. the nervous system may influence endocrine secretion and vice versa. The sources and chief physiological actions of the major endocrine hormones, and the location of the principal endocrine organs of the body are given in Table 1.1 and Figure 1.1 respectively.

The Mode of Action of Hormones on Cells

The mechanisms by which hormones exert their specific effects on target cells can be varied. Protein and polypeptide hormones do not generally penetrate into the cell interior, but react externally with a specific receptor located in the cell membrane. This may result in direct membrane effects (e.g. a change in ionic permeability or solute transport characteristics) or intracellular effects mediated by *second messenger* systems within the cell (e.g. the action of the pancreatic hormone **glucagon** on liver cell membranes to stimulate glycogenolysis, is mediated by *adenylate cyclase* and the production of *cAMP* (cyclic 3′,5′-adenosine monophosphate; Figure 1.2)). In the case of the pancreatic hormone **insulin**, the peptide is believed to interact initially with surface insulin receptors, followed by an internalization of the insulin-receptor complex and a direct modulation of key enzymatic processes (see Chapter 5).

Steroid hormones on the other hand (e.g. the sex hormones **oestradiol**, **progesterone**, **testosterone**; the adrenal corticosteroids **cortisol**, **aldosterone** and also **vitamin D**), being lipophilic, enter cells directly to combine with highly specific *receptor proteins* in the cytoplasm or the nucleus. This hormone-receptor complex then acts within the cell nucleus where it binds to special acceptor sites (*hormone*

Endocrine gland	Hormone released	Abbr.	Main actions
Hypothalamus	Gonadotrophin releasing hormone	GnRH	Stimulation of LH and FSH release
	Thyrotrophin releasing hormone	TRH	Stimulation of TSH release
	Corticotrophin releasing hormone	CRH	Stimulation of ACTH release
	Growth hormone releasing hormone	GHRH	Stimulation of GH release
	Somatostatin	SS	GH-release inhibiting factor
	Dopamine		Prolactin-release inhibiting factor
Anterior pituitary	Luteinizing hormone	LH	Development of corpus luteum; stimulation of sex hormone production
	Follicle stimulating hormone	FSH	Growth of ovarian follicles/ spermatogenesis
	Thyrotrophin	TSH	Release of thyroid hormone
	Corticotrophin	ACTH	Release of adrenocortical steroids
	Growth hormone	GH	Bone and muscle growth
	Prolactin	PRL	Milk production
Posterior pituitary*	Oxytocin		Milk ejection
	Vasopressin	AVP	Exerts antidiuretic action
Thyroid (follicles)	Thyroxine and tri-iodothyronine	T_4, T_3	Increase in basal metabolic rate (BMR)
(C-cells)	Calcitonin		Control of Ca metabolism
Parathyroid	Parathyroid hormone	PTH	Control of Ca metabolism
Adrenal cortex	Cortisol		Influences carbohydrate/protein/fat metabolism
	Aldosterone		Influences Na^+/H_2O balance
Adrenal medulla	Adrenaline Noradrenaline		Influences blood pressure/blood sugar level
Ovary (follicle)	Oestrogen		Stimulates development of female reproductive tract
(corpus luteum)	Progesterone		Maintains pregnancy; stimulates development of uterus/ mammary gland
Testes	Testosterone		Anabolism; stimulates development of male reproductive tract; spermatogenesis; libido
Pancreas (islets of Langerhans)	Insulin Glucagon		Control of carbohydrate metabolism

* Note: oxytocin and vasopressin are really hypothalamic hormones produced in the neurosecretory cells of the paraventricular (PVN) and supraoptic (SO) nuclei, and transported through the axons of their neurosecretory cells to the posterior pituitary, where they are stored and eventually released (see Chapter 2).

Table 1.1. Major endocrine glands and the principal hormones they produce.

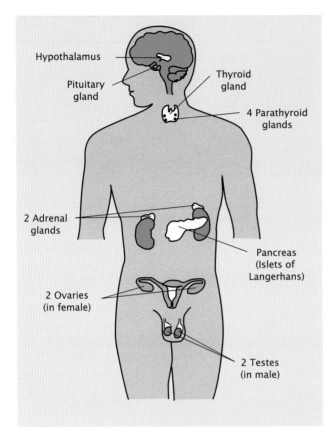

Figure 1.1. The location of principal endocrine organs in the body.

response elements) on the nuclear DNA, leading ultimately to a change in the rate of transcription of specific genes. Thyroid hormones are also able to penetrate the cell membrane (mainly by diffusion), but unlike steroids, they bind *directly* with high affinity receptor proteins associated with the nuclear DNA to influence mRNA transcription and protein synthesis (see Figures 3.5 and 4.4 respectively).

☞ cAMP is not the only second messenger that may be involved in mediating hormone actions. Other signal transduction mechanisms involving, for example, the stimulation of *guanylate cyclase* (to produce *cGMP*, cyclic 3',5'-guanosine monophosphate), or activation of *protein kinase C* (via stimulation of *phospholipase C* and hydrolysis of membrane polyphosphoinositides to yield inositol-1,4,5-trisphosphate (IP$_3$) and diacylglycerol (DAG)) may also function to control certain hormone responses.

Some hormone receptors can also mediate the breakdown of membrane phospholipids via the activation of the enzyme *phospholipase A$_2$*, resulting in the production

of *arachidonic acid* and a range of 'eicosanoid' metabolites (e.g. prostaglandins, thromboxanes, leukotrienes and platelet-activating factor (PAF)) involved in allergic responses and inflammation. Arachidonic acid itself may also function as an intracellular messenger to regulate the activity of certain enzymes (e.g. *protein kinase C*) and membrane ion channels.

Control of Hormone Secretion: The Concept of Feedback Mechanisms

In order to maintain the correct regulatory function of a hormone, the endocrine gland should receive constant feedback information about the state of the system being regulated, so that hormone release can be finely adjusted (closed-loop system).

The secretory activity of most endocrine target organs is controlled by the **anterior pituitary**, which is in turn, under the influence of **hypothalamic releasing hormones/factors** released by hypothalamic nerve fibres into the pituitary blood supply.

☞ Modulatory feedback loops also exist, that do not involve the hypothalamus and anterior pituitary e.g. in the control of **insulin** or **parathyroid hormone** release.

The principal endocrine feedback mechanisms are as follows:

Direct Negative Feedback

This is the most common 'closed-loop' control mechanism, in which an *increase* in the level of a circulating hormone, *decreases* the secretory activity of the cells producing it. The loop is illustrated schematically in Figure 1.3. In this typical hierarchical arrangement, specialized groups of nerve cells in the hypothalamus synthesize specific peptides (**releasing hormones**) that are secreted into the capillary network feeding the anterior pituitary gland, and then stimulate the pituitary cells to release specific **trophic hormones**. These peptides, in turn, stimulate their particular target gland cells to release a **target gland hormone** into the general circulation. The latter then exerts a negative feedback effect on the anterior pituitary, to regulate the level of trophic hormone release.

Example
The secretion of **thyroxine** by the thyroid gland is directly controlled by the pituitary trophic hormone **TSH (thyroid**

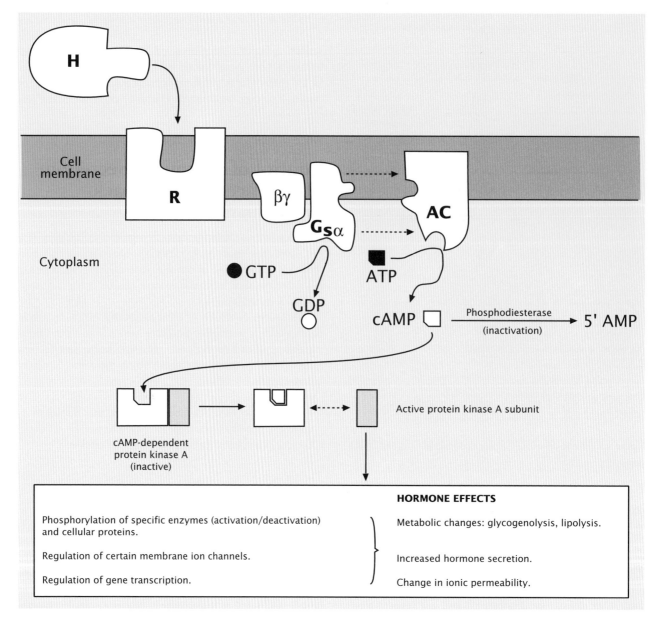

Figure 1.2. Schematic diagram showing basic mechanism by which certain hormones can influence target cell activity by stimulating the production of an intracellular second messenger (cyclic AMP). The binding of hormone to an external receptor site (R) activates an intermediate stimulatory *guanine nucleotide regulatory protein (G protein: G_s)* leading to dissociation of bound GDP (guanosine diphosphate) and association of GTP (guanosine triphosphate). The G protein α-subunit (+GTP) then dissociates to activate adenylate cyclase (AC) leading to formation of cAMP and activation of protein kinase A. Subsequent phosphorylation of specific enzymes/cellular proteins causes changes in their activity, resulting in the hormone effect. cAMP is metabolized to 5′-AMP by the enzyme phosphodiesterase. *Note:* some hormone receptors linked to an *inhibitory* G protein (G_i) can produce a *reduction* in cAMP formation.

stimulating hormone). A high blood level of thyroxine diminishes the output of TSH, so that the activity of the thyroid gland decreases (and *vice versa*). Similar feedback mechanisms govern the secretory activity of other target organs e.g. the adrenal cortex, ovaries and testes.

Indirect Negative Feedback

Here, the target gland hormone inhibits the release of pituitary trophic hormone *indirectly*, by inhibiting the secretion of hypothalamic releasing hormone. This type of mechanism appears particularly important in regula-

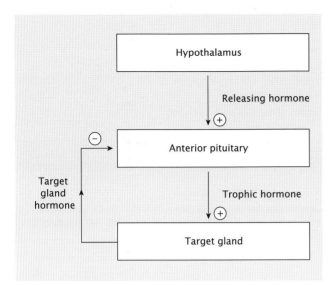

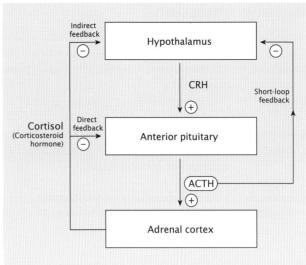

Figure 1.3. Schematic representation of a simple endocrine, direct negative feedback loop. Secretion of a specific releasing hormone by hypothalamic nerve cells, stimulates cells of the anterior pituitary to release a trophic hormone. This, in turn, initiates release of target hormone from the selected target gland. Circulating levels of target gland hormone exert a negative (inhibitory) effect on the anterior pituitary to control trophic hormone release.

Figure 1.4. Endocrine feedback loops involving direct, indirect and 'short-loop' negative feedback mechanisms. The hypothalamic-pituitary control of corticosteroid hormone production by the adrenal gland is used here as an example (see Chapter 3). Hypothalamic corticotrophin releasing hormone (CRH) stimulates the anterior pituitary to release corticotrophin (ACTH), responsible for releasing cortisol from the adrenal cortex. Cortisol inhibits ACTH release by direct negative feedback on the pituitary, and indirectly by modulating secretion of hypothalamic CRH. The trophic hormone ACTH also exerts an inhibitory effect on CRH release by a 'short-loop' feedback mechanism.

ting adrenal and gonadal (testicular and ovarian) hormone secretions.

Example

The **corticosteroid** hormones secreted by the adrenal gland may indirectly inhibit the release of **corticotrophin (adrenocorticotrophic hormone, ACTH)** from the anterior pituitary, by inhibiting the release of hypothalamic **corticotrophin releasing hormone (CRH)**. In addition, the trophic hormone itself (ACTH) may act back directly on the hypothalamic neurones to ultimately inhibit its own release (*'short-loop' feedback*) (Figure 1.4).

Positive Feedback

Such a mechanism is less common, and tends to be intrinsically unstable, as it attempts to *increase* rather than stabilize the level of a circulating hormone. A hormone may either facilitate its own release directly, by acting on the anterior pituitary, or indirectly by stimulating hypothalamic hormone release.

Example

During the female menstrual cycle, a positive feedback loop is activated when the blood level of **oestrogen**, released from the ovaries, attains a certain high threshold level. At this point, oestrogen *stimulates* (rather than inhibits) the *pulsatile* release of the **gonadotrophic hormones, luteinizing hormone (LH)** and **follicle stimulating hormone (FSH)** from the pituitary, and also the hypothalamic **gonadotrophin releasing hormone, (GnRH)**. The resultant surge in gonadotrophin secretion (particularly LH) leads to *ovulation* and abrupt termination of the positive feedback loop (see Chapter 6). ■

Review Questions

Question 1:   *Define the terms* exocrine, endocrine, paracrine *and* hormone.

Question 2:   *State the three main chemical groups of hormones.*

Question 3:   *Outline the basic mechanisms by which hormones exert their effects on target cells.*

Question 4:   *Give examples of some signal transduction mechanisms that may be involved in mediating hormone actions.*

Question 5:   *Explain the principle of* hormonal feedback.

Question 6:   *Explain the functional relation between the hypothalamus and anterior pituitary in controlling hormone release.*

Question 7:   *Describe (giving examples) the various types of hormonal feedback mechanism.*

Question 8:   *Draw a diagram showing the location of the principal endocrine organs in the body.*

References

- **Goodman HM.** (1988). Introduction. In *Basic Medical Endocrinology*, Raven Press, New York, pp. 1–25

- **Hedge GA, Colb HD, Goodman RL.** (1987). General principles of endocrinology. In *Clinical Endocrine Physiology*, WB Saunders Co., Philadelphia, pp. 3–33

- **Guyton AC, Hall JE.** (1996). Introduction to endocrinology. In *Textbook of Medical Physiology*, 9th ed. WB Saunders Company, USA, pp. 925–932

- **Thibodeau GA, Patton KT.** (1993). The endocrine system. In *Anatomy & Physiology*, 2nd ed. Mosby-Year Book, Inc., USA, pp. 402–439

2 The Hypothalamus and Pituitary

Structure and Histology

The secretions of the hypothalamus and anterior pituitary play a major role in the control of hormone release from other endocrine glands.

The **hypothalamus** is situated in part of the forebrain known as the **diencephalon**, located between the cerebrum (*telencephalon*) and the midbrain (*mesencephalon*); it lies immediately beneath the thalamus, forming the floor and lower lateral walls of the third ventricle. Although it is a relatively small area of the brain, it performs many important functions e.g. controlling eating, drinking and sexual drives/behaviour, as well as essential autonomic nervous activities (regulation of blood pressure and heart rate). It is also involved in the maintenance of body temperature, controlling the sleep-wake cycle and for setting emotional states such as fear, pain, anger and pleasure.

Specialized clusters of neurones within the *supraoptic* and *paraventricular nuclei* of the hypothalamus have a vital *neuroendocrine* function in synthesizing the peptide hormones **vasopressin** and **oxytocin**, which are transported down their axons and released from the *posterior pituitary* to affect water balance and uterine contractility/breast milk ejection respectively. Other hypothalamic neurones secrete *releasing* or *inhibiting hormones* into the blood, which influence the secretion of *trophic hormones* by the anterior pituitary gland (discussed below); the hypothalamus thus represents a major link between the nervous and endocrine systems.

The **pituitary gland** is a dual organ (about 1 cm in diameter), located in a bony hollow at the base of the brain (just below the hypothalamus), to which it is linked by the *pituitary (infundibular) stalk*. It is formed embryologically from oral (epithelial) and neural (hypothalamic) ectoderm fusing to form the anterior lobe (*pars distalis*; ca. 75% of the pituitary mass) and posterior lobe (*neurohypophysis* or *pars nervosa*) respectively (Figure 2.1); these two parts function as independent endocrine glands. In some vertebrate species (e.g. fish, reptiles and amphibians) a distinct intermediate lobe of endocrine tissue (*pars intermedia*) is present as part of the *adenohypophysis*; this portion of the pituitary secretes the peptide hormone **melanocyte stimulating hormone (MSH)**, important in controlling skin pigmentation changes

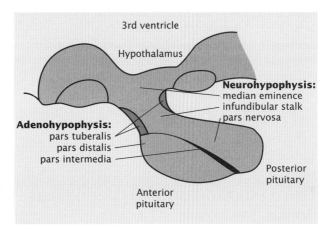

Figure 2.1. Diagram showing basic anatomical features of the pituitary gland, divided into functionally-independent anterior (adenohypophysis) and posterior (neurohypophysis) portions and connected to the hypothalamus by the infundibular stalk. The *pars intermedia* (intermediate lobe) is not well developed in man.

(see below). In adult humans, the intermediate lobe is not well developed, and exists only in vestigial form.

The anterior pituitary secretes *six* principal peptides, known as **trophic hormones**. With the exception of **growth hormone (GH)** and **prolactin (PRL)**, all have their major effects restricted to specific target organs.

Hormone		Target organ(s)
FSH, LH	(Gonadotrophins)	Gonads (ovaries/testes)
ACTH	(Corticotrophin)	Adrenal gland
TSH	(Thyrotrophin)	Thyroid gland
PRL	(Prolactin)	Mammary gland
GH	(Somatotrophin)	Bone, soft tissue, viscera
Mnemonic: "F — L — A — T — PRo — G"		

Histology

The secretory cells of the anterior pituitary may be classified according to the trophic hormone they release, and their cytoplasmic staining characteristics; different cells may also be identified by more specific immunocytochemical methods, using selective hormone antisera, or by *in situ* hybridization techniques, which detect the expression of the corresponding hormone genes. The various cell-types and the hormones they release may be summarized as follows:

1. *Somatotrophs*   Secrete Growth Hormone (GH)
2. *Mammotrophs*   Secrete Prolactin (PRL)
3. *Corticotrophs*   Secrete Corticotrophin (ACTH)
4. *Thyrotrophs*   Secrete Thyrotrophin (TSH)
5. *Gonadotrophs*   Secrete Gonadotrophins (LH/FSH)

☞ Some gonadotroph cells may secrete *both* LH and FSH.

The Hypothalamic-Hypophyseal Portal System

Synthesis and release of these trophic hormones is determined partly by direct feedback effects exerted by the target gland hormones (Chapter 1), and partly by specific *hypothalamic releasing or inhibiting hormones*. These agents are secreted by specialized hypothalamic (peptidergic) neurones with nerve endings in the region of the *median eminence*. The *hypothalamic-hypophyseal portal system of veins*, takes blood from a primary capillary bed in the median eminence, along the pituitary stalk, and enters the anterior pituitary to form a secondary bed of capillaries; the released hypothalamic hormones readily enter the portal capillaries and are then transported via the portal veins to the anterior lobe, where they exert their effects (Figure 2.2).

Hypothalamic Releasing and Inhibiting Hormones that Influence the Anterior Pituitary

The actions of the principal hypothalamic hormones, and their current therapeutic uses may be summarized as follows:

Gonadotrophin Releasing Hormone

Gonadotrophin releasing hormone (GnRH), (also known as *luteinizing hormone releasing hormone (LHRH)* or **gonadorelin**) is a linear decapeptide, that is released in a pulsatile fashion from hypothalamic GnRH neurones.

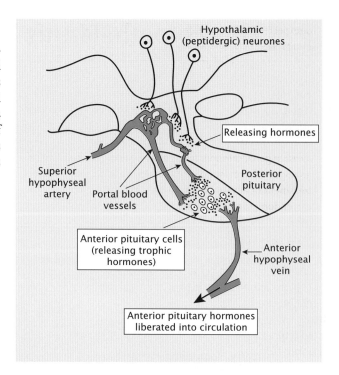

Figure 2.2. The hypothalamic-hypophyseal portal system. Hypothalamic peptidergic neurones secrete releasing hormones that are transported by small hypophyseal portal blood vessels in the median eminence and pituitary stalk, to affect target cells of the anterior pituitary. These respond by releasing trophic hormones that enter into the pituitary venous blood supply and are carried to target tissues via the general circulation.

Although other hypothalamic and/or gonadal peptides may be involved, both luteinizing hormone (LH) and follicle stimulating hormone (FSH) release is most likely promoted by a single releasing hormone (GnRH), whose production can be inhibited by circulating *oestrogens* (indirect negative feedback). This phenomenon may largely underlie the effectiveness of the 'combined' oral contraceptive pill (see Chapter 6).

Synthetic gonadorelin *(Fertiral)* is available in the form of an injection (500 μg/ml) given intravenously or by pulsatile subcutaneous injection for the treatment of infertility and amenorrhoea (cessation of menstruation) in women, induction of puberty or for assessment of pituitary function.

☞ Because of the very short half-life of GnRH in the circulation, there has been considerable interest in modifying the GnRH molecule to produce stable analogues that may be more suitable for clinical applications. A number of synthetic analogues such as **buserelin**, **goserelin**, **leuprorelin** or **nafarelin**, with potent GnRH activity (agonistic analogues) have been developed, but their clinical testing revealed unexpected *inhibitory* rather than stimulatory effects on the pituitary-gonadal axis, when given continuously. Thus, after initial stimulation of gonadotrophin release, the prolonged (2–4 week) administration of these agents (by subcutaneous injection or nasal spray), ultimately causes a down-regulation and loss of GnRH receptors from the pituitary gonadotrophs, a reduced responsiveness to further stimulation by GnRH (or agonistic GnRH analogues) and a *decrease* in gonadotrophin (and gonadal steroid) release. GnRH analogues have found clinical application mainly in the treatment of advanced, androgen-dependent prostatic cancer, endometriosis (see Chapter 6), precocious puberty and other conditions where suppression of gonadotrophin release is desirable.

Analogues of GnRH which bind competitively to GnRH receptors but do not exhibit GnRH agonist activity (GnRH antagonists) have also been developed; their early clinical usage was however, complicated by local skin reactions (reddening, oedema) at the site of injection, due to a histamine-releasing action. Some of the recently synthesized GnRH antagonist analogues are devoid of these untoward side effects, and show considerable promise for future use in the control of fertility and for other clinical applications where pituitary suppression of GnRH action is required.

Corticotrophin Releasing Hormone

Corticotrophin releasing hormone (corticoliberin, CRH) (also referred to as *corticotrophin releasing factor, CRF*) is a 41 amino acid peptide, responsible for controlling the secretion of *corticotrophin (ACTH)*. This action can be influenced by several other substances: in particular, glucocorticoid hormones *(Chapter 3)*, that inhibit the releasing effect of CRH on the pituitary corticotrophs (may be important in negative feedback control), and **vasopressin**, **oxytocin** (see p. 16–17), or **adrenaline** which potentiate it. Various endogenous neurotransmitters are also involved in the regulation of hypothalamic CRH release: e.g. *acetylcholine* and *serotonin* (5-hydroxytryptamine; 5-HT) directly facilitate its release, whereas the inhibitory amino acid GABA (*γ-aminobutyric acid*), *dopamine* and *noradrenaline* have release-inhibitory effects. Glucocorticoids may also inhibit the release of CRH at the hypothalamic level (*indirect negative feedback*). The CRH receptor on the pituitary cells appears to be linked to the adenylate cyclase second messenger system.

Thyrotrophin Releasing Hormone

Thyrotrophin releasing hormone (TRH) was the first hypothalamic factor to be isolated and characterized. It is a simple tripeptide (*pyroGlu-His-Pro-NH₂*), and is particularly potent in promoting the release of *thyrotrophin (TSH)* (picogram quantities are effective). TRH also promotes the secretion of pituitary *prolactin*. Interestingly, TRH may be found elsewhere throughout the brain and spinal cord (where it may act as a neuromodulator or transmitter) and also in the gastrointestinal tract and pancreas, although its functions here are uncertain. Synthetic **TRH** (*Protirelin*) is available for clinical use (by intravenous injection) in thyroid function tests.

Prolactin-Releasing/Inhibiting Factors

Although TRH is believed to be an important hypothalamic prolactin-releasing factor, prolactin can also be released by several other endogenous peptides e.g. *oxytocin, vasoactive intestinal polypeptide (VIP), angiotensin-II, substance P, galanin* and *neurotensin*. The prolactin release-*inhibiting* factor however, is a simple non-peptide, *dopamine*, that is released into the portal blood supply by specific dopaminergic neurones originating in the hypothalamus. This tonic inhibitory action of dopamine, effectively maintains prolactin secretion at a minimal level, until required during lactation, or release in response to stress.

☞ About 70% of hypothalamic prolactin release-inhibiting activity can be attributed to dopamine, while the remaining 30% can be accounted for by other factors including **GnRH-associated peptide (GAP)**. GAP is a 56 amino acid peptide derived from the GnRH precursor protein (proGnRH), that is believed to be co-produced with GnRH in the same population of hypothalamic neurones and co-secreted into the pituitary portal blood to affect prolactin release.

Growth Hormone Releasing Hormone

Growth hormone releasing hormone (GHRH) (**somatocrinin**) is a 44 amino acid peptide (derived from a larger precursor molecule) that is responsible for stimulating (specifically) the synthesis and release of pituitary **growth hormone** (GH). It is the 1-21 N terminal fragment of the molecule that appears to be necessary for biological activity. Although GHRH bears a strong structural resemblance to the pancreatic hormone *glucagon*, and is also known to be present in the pancreas and upper intestinal tract, its physiological functions outside the brain remain uncertain. A synthetic analogue of GHRH, **sermorelin** (*Geref 50*) (administered by intravenous injection) is now available for use as a diagnostic test for normal pituitary secretion of GH (see also below: the *insulin tolerance test*). Other small peptide and non-peptide derivatives have also recently been developed which show potent GH-releasing properties (*GH secretagogues*, e.g. **hexarelin**) and may eventually prove useful for the treatment of short-stature children with abnormal GH secretion. Interestingly, these agents appear to stimulate the pituitary in synergy with GHRH, although they interact with a different type of receptor.

A hypothalamic GH-release *inhibiting* hormone, **somatostatin (SS)** (often referred to as **somatotrophin release inhibiting hormone, SRIH**) has also been characterized and synthesized. It is a cyclic 14 amino acid peptide, with a powerful, receptor mediated (non-competitive), inhibitory effect on the action of GHRH on anterior pituitary somatotrophs; it is also capable of inhibiting the basal secretion of *TSH* and *prolactin* from the pituitary gland. SS can be found elsewhere in the brain and spinal cord, the gastrointestinal tract (myenteric plexus), and in the pancreas, where it suppresses the release of both insulin and glucagon. A stable, long-acting analogue of SS, **octreotide** (*Sandostatin*), is available as a therapeutic agent (given by subcutaneous injection) in the short-term treatment of *acromegaly* (see p. 15), and some hypersecretory endocrine tumours (e.g. insulinomas, glucagonomas and VIPomas).

☞ VIP (vasoactive intestinal polypeptide; 28 amino acid residues), is a member of the secretin-glucagon family of peptides, found throughout the gastrointestinal tract (mainly the pancreas and neurones of the duodenum) and also in the brain (hypothalamus and cerebral cortex). Patients with abnormally high plasma levels of VIP arising from VIP-secreting tumours, can suffer from severe watery diarrhoea and electrolyte imbalance.

Hormones of the Anterior Pituitary

Gonadotrophins

Gonadotrophins are complex glycoprotein (carbohydrate-containing) hormones of around 28 kDa molecular weight. They each consist of two glycoprotein subunits α and β, with the β sequence being different for LH and FSH respectively. The common α subunit appears to be necessary for the interaction of the gonadotrophins with their target gland receptors.

LUTEINIZING HORMONE (LH)

In *females*, a surge of LH (in co-operation with FSH) at midcycle, induces ovulation, then maintains the *corpus luteum* after ovulation; (this secretes **progesterone**). In *males*, it stimulates the interstitial (*Leydig*) cells in the testes to produce **testosterone**.

Control of release is primarily via hypothalamic GnRH (pulsatile), and modulated by feedback loops involving the ovarian or testicular steroids. The **human chorionic gonadotrophin (hCG)**, produced by the placenta during pregnancy, has a similar structure to LH, and exhibits LH-like activity.

FOLLICLE STIMULATING HORMONE (FSH)

This hormone (along with LH) promotes the development of the ovarian follicle (and consequent **oestrogen** production) and stimulates spermatogenesis in males.

Recombinant FSH (*Puregon*) is now available for treatment of anovulatory infertility in women undergoing assisted conception.

Control of release: is principally via GnRH, and also shows a pulsatile pattern (less marked than that of LH). In the *male*, FSH also stimulates the *Sertoli cells* of the testes to produce a peptide, **inhibin** which provides the main direct negative feedback control of FSH biosynthesis and release from the anterior pituitary. It has little or no effect on LH release. In the female, a similar peptide released by *granulosa cells* of the developing ovarian follicle, appears to serve a similar inhibitory function on FSH secretion. Inhibin may also have an important intragonadal (paracrine) function in enhancing the LH-stimulated production of testicular and ovarian steroids (see Chapter 6) (Figure 2.3).

Hyposecretion of gonadotrophins leads to amenorrhoea, sterility and loss of sexual potency. In the young, the sex organs and secondary sexual characteristics fail to develop (delayed puberty).

Hypersecretion of FSH and LH is extremely rare, but in children it could lead to sexual precocity (excessive premature development).

Thyrotrophin (Thyroid Stimulating Hormone, TSH)

Like the gonadotrophins, this glycoprotein hormone consists of two polypeptide chains, α and β, with the α chain being identical to that found in LH, FSH and hCG. Its primary action is to stimulate the thyroid gland to secrete the thyroid hormones **tri-iodothyronine (T_3)** and **thyroxine (T_4)**. This is achieved by:

1. Stimulation of thyroid iodide uptake;
2. Increased synthesis of the thyroidal storage protein, **thyroglobulin**;
3. Stimulation of T_3/T_4 synthesis and release, and
4. An increase in the thickness of the follicular epithelium and vascularity of the thyroid gland. Excess TSH can result in an enlarged thyroid (*goitre*).

Control of release is via hypothalamic TRH. TSH release is also influenced by circulating thyroid hormones at the pituitary level (direct negative feedback) and by some other circulating endocrine hormones e.g. cortisol, growth hormone and oestrogens. The hypothalamic factors

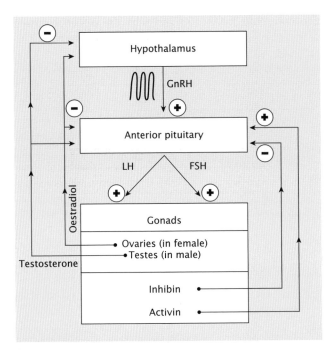

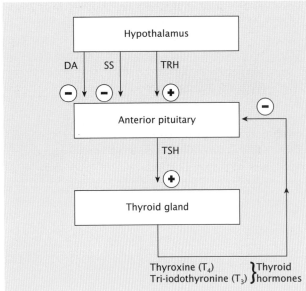

Figure 2.3. Control of gonadotrophin (LH, FSH) and gonadal steroid secretion by the hypothalamus and anterior pituitary. Pulsatile release of GnRH by the hypothalamus induces release of LH and FSH from the pituitary, that stimulate the ovaries (in the female) to produce oestradiol and progesterone, and the testes (in the male) to produce testosterone; these steroids exert negative feedback control of GnRH and LH release at the hypothalamic and pituitary levels. Secretion of FSH is controlled mainly by feedback loops involving the gonadal peptides inhibin and activin.

somatostatin and *dopamine* exert some tonic inhibitory influence on TSH secretion (Figure 2.4). The normal plasma level of TSH is within the range 0.5–5 µU/ml (about 10 pM).

Hyposecretion produces a clinical picture similar to primary thyroid deficiency.

Hypersecretion gives the symptoms of hyperthyroidism similar to *Graves' disease* (see Chapter 4).

Corticotrophin (Adrenocorticotrophic Hormone, ACTH)

This single-chain peptide hormone consists of 39 amino acids and is derived from a larger precursor molecule, *preproopiomelanocortin (POMC)*. It stimulates the adrenal cortex to secrete *glucocorticoids* (mainly **cortisol**) and also small amounts of sex hormones (androgens and oestrogens); this action is mediated by specific high affinity ACTH receptors present on the adrenal cell membrane, linked to intracellular production of cAMP. The synthetic preparation **tetracosactrin** (*Syncathen*) containing the first 24 amino

Figure 2.4. Regulation of pituitary thyrotrophin (TSH) secretion via release of hypothalamic TRH and by direct negative feedback effects of the thyroid gland hormones T_3 and T_4 on the anterior pituitary. Dopamine (DA) and somatostatin (SS) released by specific hypothalamic neurones, also exert a tonic inhibitory action on pituitary TSH release.

acid sequence of ACTH, may be given by intramuscular or intravenous injection to test adrenocortical function.

☞ Several other peptide fragments derived from the POMC prohormone are also released from the pituitary along with ACTH during stress; in particular, β-**lipotrophin (β-LPH)** and β-**endorphin** (Figure 2.5). Beta-endorphin belongs to the class of endogenous opioid compounds that are normally produced by the brain and other tissues, and bind to the same receptors which interact with morphine, heroin and other opioid drugs. Endogenous opioids produced in the CNS are believed to exert anti-nociceptive and pain-reducing effects. However, the hormonal role (if any) of these peptides produced in the pituitary, has not been fully established. In reptiles and amphibia, further processing of ACTH or γ-**lipotrophin** within the intermediate lobe of the pituitary (*pars intermedia*; not well developed in humans) can occur to yield α- or β- forms of the **melanocyte stimulating hormone (MSH).** This peptide acts on the skin melanocytes to disperse melanin pigment, and therefore to induce darkening of the skin (important for camouflage). In view of the structural overlap between ACTH and MSH, the former can, *in excess amounts*, exert MSH-like activity. Interestingly, POMC and POMC-derived peptides are also produced locally in the skin by melanocytes and keratinocytes, and may therefore be important for maintaining normal skin functions.

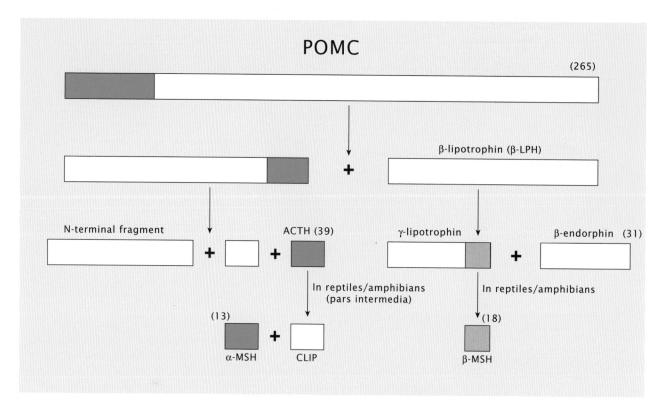

Figure 2.5. Peptide hormone fragments derived from the sequential proteolysis of the precursor molecule (prohormone) preproopiomelanocortin (POMC) in the anterior pituitary gland. In certain reptiles and amphibians, corticotrophin (ACTH) can be further processed by cells of the *pars intermedia* to produce α-MSH (comprising the first 13 amino acids of ACTH) and γ-lipotrophin can be cleaved to yield β-MSH (melanocyte stimulating hormones). CLIP is a corticotrophin-like intermediate lobe peptide. Numbers in brackets indicate length of amino acid chains.

Control of release is mainly via hypothalamic CRH, and regulated by circulating cortisol (direct and indirect negative feedback) (Figure 2.6). Pharmacological inhibition of release can also be produced by administration of synthetic corticosteroid analogues. ACTH secretion shows a characteristic circadian rhythm (low level around midnight-peak at around 6 a.m.). Release of ACTH (and POMC cleavage products) is promoted by *stress* e.g. trauma, pain, fear or hypoglycaemia (low blood sugar level) and also by the posterior pituitary peptide *vasopressin*. The latter may, in fact, act synergistically with CRH to regulate ACTH release from pituitary cells.

Hyposecretion of ACTH (rare) causes failure of cortisol secretion, a general lack of health and well being, a reduced response to stress and skin depigmentation.

Hypersecretion (due to a pituitary microadenoma, or 'ectopic' non-endocrine tumour) will result in *Cushing's syndrome* (Chapter 3). When Cushing's syndrome arises due to a pituitary tumour, it is called *Cushing's disease,* which nowadays is treated either by surgical (trans-sphenoidal)

removal of the adenoma (where possible), or by external pituitary irradiation therapy. Alternatively, where surgery is inappropriate, patients may be treated with **aminoglutethimide** (*Orimeten*) an *aromatase enzyme inhibitor* which also interferes with adrenal steroid synthesis; maintenance doses of a glucocorticoid (e.g. *hydrocortisone*; Chapter 3) may also need to be given in this case. [The use of aromatase inhibitors in the treatment of advanced breast or prostate cancer is discussed in Chapter 6].

Under certain circumstances, treatment may involve bilateral adrenalectomy (removal of the adrenal glands). However, following this, the negative feedback effect of cortisol on the pituitary tumour is lost, allowing it to grow further and secrete more ACTH, resulting in excess skin pigmentation (a symptom of *Nelson's syndrome*).

☞ A patient that has undergone total adrenalectomy will require lifelong supplements of adrenal steroids (glucocorticoids and mineralocorticoids; Chapter 3) to remain alive and healthy.

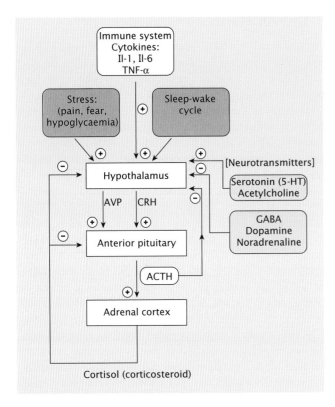

Figure 2.6. Control of pituitary corticotrophin (ACTH) release by hypothalamic releasing hormone (CRH) and negative feedback loops involving the adrenal corticosteroid cortisol, acting back on the anterior pituitary and hypothalamus. The secretion of CRH by the hypothalamus is primarily influenced by various stressful stimuli (e.g. acute trauma, pain, fear, or hypoglycaemia), by the sleep-wake cycle, and also by endogenous neurotransmitters (5-HT and acetylcholine facilitate CRH release, whereas GABA, dopamine and noradrenaline have an inhibitory effect). Arginine-vasopressin (AVP) secreted by the hypothalamus, is a powerful stimulus of pituitary ACTH release. ACTH itself can inhibit CRH release by a negative feedback effect on the hypothalamus ('short-loop' feedback). Various *cytokines*, including *interleukins (IL-1, IL-6)* and *tumour necrosis factor-α (TNF-α)* released by macrophages, monocytes, endothelial cells and lymphocytes during inflammatory/immune responses, have a direct stimulatory effect on hypothalamic CRH and pituitary ACTH release (see Chapter 3).

Prolactin

Prolactin (PRL) is a single chain peptide (198 amino acids) with a chemical structure very similar to that of *growth hormone (GH)*. It is principally involved (in co-operation with other hormones) in the development of the female breast, and in the initiation and maintenance of lactation (milk production) shortly after childbirth. It is released from pituitary mammotroph cells in increasing amounts during pregnancy (under the influence of circulating *oestrogen*), and acutely in response to suckling, by means of a sensory neural reflex arising in the nipple. The suckling reflex also depends on a prior 'sensitization' of the secretory alveoli of the breast by oestrogen. Although its function in human males is unknown, excess prolactin levels can exert powerful inhibitory effects on both male and female gonadal function and libido (sexual drive), primarily via actions on the CNS and by suppression of GnRH release.

Control of release is via (non-specific) hypothalamic inhibiting and releasing factors. The dominant tonic influence is *inhibitory* via release of hypothalamic **dopamine**, from dopaminergic neurones, into the portal circulation. The dopamine receptor agonist **bromocriptine** can thus be effective in controlling excessive prolactin secretion. Release is *promoted* by various substances including TRH, VIP and also by various stresses e.g. fear, hypoglycaemia, or anaesthesia/ surgery. The posterior pituitary peptide *oxytocin* is also a powerful releasing agent, and may be involved in the suckling-induced response. Prolactin exerts a stimulatory short-loop feedback effect on the hypothalamic dopamine-secreting neurones, thereby inhibiting its own release (Figure 2.7). Like ACTH, plasma levels of prolactin show a distinct circadian rhythm (highest level at night) in both males and non-pregnant females; this rhythm disappears during pregnancy and lactation, when prolactin release is at its highest.

Hyposecretion of prolactin leads to failure of lactation in women.

Hypersecretion of prolactin (*hyperprolactinaemia*) may result from a pituitary tumour (prolactinoma; one of the most common type of pituitary tumour) or hypothalamic disease. Infertility and menstrual complaints are the principal symptoms; in men, this manifests as a decreased libido, inadequate sperm production and impotence, whereas in women, there may be a complete lack of menstruation. Overproduction of prolactin may also lead to inappropriate (non-pregnant) milk production (*galactorrhoea*). The latter condition may also occur when hypothalamic dopamine action is antagonized by therapeutic administration of certain antidepressants and tranquillizers such as the *phenothiazine* **trifluoperazine** (*Stelazine*) or the *butyrophenone* **haloperidol** (*Serenace*) prescribed for psychiatric disorders.

The effects of excess prolactin secretion on gonadal function is believed to result from (a) an indirect inhibition of LH/FSH release by blocking the synthesis and release of hypothalamic GnRH and (b) a direct inhibition of LH/FSH action on the ovaries and testes.

☞ There is a tendency for ovulation to be inhibited during the period of breast feeding, although this inhibition is by no means reliable.

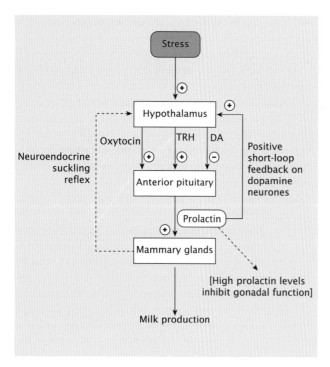

Figure 2.7. Control of prolactin secretion by hypothalamic releasing/inhibiting factors. The principal prolactin-releasing hormones are TRH (thyrotrophin releasing hormone) and oxytocin (released during the infant suckling response); release is also promoted by various stress factors. Secretion of dopamine (DA) by specific hypothalamic neurones, exerts a tonic inhibitory influence on pituitary prolactin release. Prolactin itself can inhibit its own release by *stimulating* hypothalamic dopamine production (positive short-loop feedback). Excessively high levels of prolactin can inhibit gonadal function.

Treatment. This may be directed at the underlying tumour (surgical removal or radiotherapy) or by oral administration of the dopamine D_2 receptor *agonist* **bromocriptine** (*Parlodel*) (1–10 mg daily), which should reduce the plasma prolactin concentration and tumour size, and eventually restore gonadal function back to normal. This drug is also used to suppress unwanted lactation after childbirth and in the treatment of *acromegaly* (see below) and cyclical benign breast disorders.

Two other more selective and longer-acting dopamine D_2 agonists, **cabergoline** (*Dostinex*) and **quinagolide** (*Norprolac*) have recently been introduced, with actions and uses similar to those of bromocriptine. A sustained-release injectable form of bromocriptine (*Parlodel-LAR*; given by intramuscular injection) is also currently under clinical investigation for the medical treatment of large (>10 mm) prolactin-secreting *macroprolactinomas* (associated with severe visual impairment) and also *microprolactinomas* (<10 mm size).

Growth Hormone

Growth hormone **(GH; somatotrophin)** is the most abundant of the pituitary trophic hormones, but unlike them, it can influence a variety of target tissues. It is a single chain peptide containing 191 amino acids and 2 disulphide bridges. GH promotes linear growth of bone (particularly long bones) by stimulating the growth and calcification of the epiphyseal cartilage cells; it also influences the growth of the visceral organs, adipose and connective tissue, endocrine glands and striated muscle. GH levels are at their highest during early childhood and particularly at puberty (it is essential for normal gonadal development), then levels steadily decline throughout life, implying that GH may not be essential for normal adult health. However, some recent findings suggest that GH deficiency may be responsible for some symptoms of ageing, and treatment of elderly individuals with GH has been reported to exert beneficial effects on body composition and bone density. Overproduction of GH in the young results in abnormal body growth (*gigantism*). GH also *antagonizes* the peripheral action of insulin (increases blood glucose levels) and is therefore generally considered to be a *diabetogenic* hormone; (patients suffering from GH excess can thus show a mild *hyperglycaemia* and insulin resistance).

The principal effects of GH on protein, carbohydrate and lipid metabolism are:

1. Stimulation of cellular amino acid uptake and protein synthesis (particularly in skeletal muscle and liver).
2. Stimulation of lipolysis within adipose tissue, and consequent increase in plasma free fatty acid levels.
3. Decreased glucose uptake by muscle and adipose tissue.
4. Increased gluconeogenesis (glucose output) within the liver.

Many of the actions of GH on bone and peripheral soft tissue growth are mediated *indirectly* by the GH-induced production of growth-promoting peptides known as **insulin-like growth factors (IGFs)**, derived mainly from the liver and kidney, (or produced locally) and transported in the plasma in association with specific binding proteins. The principal IGF (**IGF-1** or **somatomedin-C**) is a highly conserved 70 amino acid peptide with a close structural resemblance to the insulin precursor molecule **proinsulin** (Chapter 5). Specific receptors for IGF-1 (similar to the insulin receptor) are known to be present on skeletal muscle, liver, adipose and cartilage (chondrocyte) cells, and ultimately mediate an increase in DNA synthesis and cell division in these tissues. GH can also act *directly* on some tissues (e.g. skeletal muscle and adipose tissue) to modulate cell growth, by interacting with specific GH receptors in the target cell membrane.

Control of release (pulsatile) is via the hypothalamic releasing hormone GHRH and the release inhibiting hor-

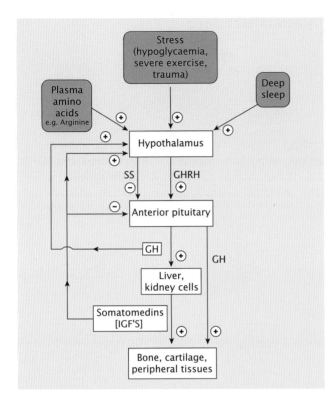

Figure 2.8. Regulation of growth hormone (GH) release. The two main hypothalamic hormones involved in the control of GH secretion are GHRH (stimulatory) and somatostatin (SS; inhibitory). GH release is also promoted by stress (particularly hypoglycaemia or exercise), deep sleep, and by some dietary amino acids. Somatomedins produced by the action of GH on liver and kidney cells, inhibit GH release via negative feedback on the pituitary and via *stimulation* of SS release from the hypothalamus. GH can also decrease its own production by *stimulating* hypothalamic SS release (positive short-loop feedback). Some actions of GH on cell growth are mediated *directly* via specific GH receptors in the target tissues.

mone somatostatin (SS) (see p. 10). Release is also promoted by stress (e.g. hypoglycaemia, cold, surgery or severe exercise), during the onset of deep sleep, and following a rise in blood levels of certain amino acids, particularly *arginine or leucine*. The response to exercise is greater in women than in men, most likely due to an enhancing effect of circulating oestrogens on GH secretion. Since GH has no specific target gland, there is no feedback control by a target gland hormone as such; GH may, however, affect its own release my means of short-loop feedback on the hypothalamus to stimulate SS secretion (see Chapter 1). Somatomedins can also affect GH release by inhibiting the action of GHRH at the pituitary level, and also indirectly, by promoting the synthesis and release of SS from the hypothalamus (Figure 2.8).

☞ In the *insulin tolerance test* of normal pituitary function, an intravenous injection of soluble insulin (0.1 U/kg) is given (under close medical supervision) to lower blood glucose to ≤40 mg/dl, and therefore to stimulate GH release. This response is reduced or lacking in patients with pronounced pituitary disorders. Measurement of serum IGF-1 levels is also a good marker of overall GH secretion. The hypoglycaemic stress test can also be used to assess the normal pituitary release of ACTH. A general insufficiency of the anterior pituitary gland is referred to as *panhypopituitarism*.

Hyposecretion

In childhood (caused by hypothalamic or pituitary dysfunction) this leads to impairment of growth (*dwarfism*), characterized by a short stature, obesity and hypoglycaemia.

Treatment. Dwarfism may be treated by initiating human GH replacement therapy (very expensive!); the authentic human hormone **somatropin** is nowadays prepared biosynthetically in bacteria by recombinant DNA technology (*Humatrope*) and administered on a body weight basis (0.5–0.7 i.u./kg) by regular subcutaneous injection over a few years. The use of GH derived from human cadaver pituitaries has therefore been discontinued (also due to risk of prion particle transmission of Creutzfeldt-Jakob disease, a form of presenile dementia). In some rare cases, dwarfism (Laron-type) can also result from an inadequate production of the IGF polypeptides in response to normal plasma levels of GH (a form of GH resistance); such individuals would not be expected to respond to exogenous GH administration, but could be treated by giving intravenous or subcutaneous doses of IGF-1.

Hypersecretion

This usually results from a benign pituitary tumour (adenoma); (ectopic release of GH or GHRH from other neuroendocrine tumours can also occur in some rare instances). *In young patients*, this leads to *gigantism*, due to excessive growth in the long bones (highest recorded giant — 8′ 11″ at 22 years). Such children tend to be tall with long arms and legs, but are physically weak.

In adults, the long bones do not grow in length; however, abnormal bone and soft tissue growth leads to coarse facial features (prominent brow, large nose, protruding jaw, enlarged lips and tongue), enlarged fleshy 'spade-like' hands and feet, and overgrowth of the soft internal organs (particularly the heart and kidneys): such patients may also be diabetic. The condition is referred to as *acromegaly,* and can develop slowly over a period of years; gradual enlargement of the pituitary tumour may also eventually lead to headaches and visual field disturbances. Plasma IGF-1 is clearly elevated in most patients.

☞ In the *glucose suppression test* for acromegaly, the patient is given 50–100 g of glucose syrup after an overnight fast, and the plasma GH level measured after 60 min. In a normally-responding individual, the increased glucose load would decrease the GH level to ≤5 ng/ml; a maintained high level (≥10 ng/ml) would however, be diagnostic of GH hypersecretion.

Treatment. This includes surgical (trans-sphenoidal or transfrontal) removal of the pituitary tumour and/or radio-therapy (less preferred). For mild cases, the dopamine receptor agonist **bromocriptine** (*Parlodel*) given orally (10–20 mg daily, for life; see p. 13) may be effective in lowering GH levels; nausea, constipation and nasal congestion are, however, common side effects with this drug, which may limit its long-term tolerability. Bromocriptine may also be used to treat persistent symptoms following irradiation therapy.

Treatment (expensive!) of acromegalic patients with the synthetic somatostatin analogue **octreotide** (*Sandostatin; 0.1–0.2 mg given subcutaneously, 3–4 times daily*) to reduce GH hypersecretion and tumour size, can be useful prior to surgical intervention. The development of long-acting depot preparations of somatostatin in the near future, should hopefully improve the medical management of this condition.

Hormones of the Posterior Pituitary

The posterior pituitary (*neurohypophysis*) does not synthe-size hormones, but it contains a large number of unmye-linated nerve fibres originating from neuronal cell bodies located within the *supraoptic (SON)* and *paraventricular (PVN)* nuclei of the hypothalamus. These fibres form the *hypothalamo-hypophyseal tract within the pituitary stalk*. These neurones synthesize (predominantly) two nonapeptide (nine amino acid) hormones, **vasopressin** and **oxytocin** respec-tively, which are then transported as protein (*neurophysin*)-bound secretory granules down the nerve fibres, to collect at the nerve terminals within the posterior pituitary. The hormones are released by exocytosis into the capillary blood-stream running close to the nerve terminal swellings (Fig-ure 2.9). The posterior pituitary gland also contains numerous non-secretory neuroglial cells (*pituicytes*) scat-tered among the nerve fibres.

Vasopressin

The principal action of **vasopressin** (also called arginine vasopressin, AVP) is to stimulate the reabsorption of water from the distal convoluted tubules and collecting ducts of

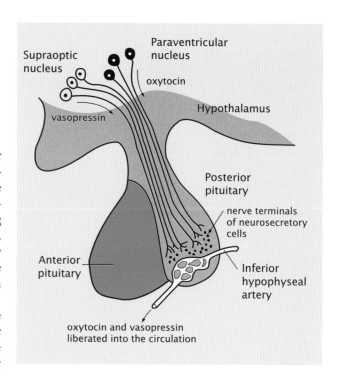

Figure 2.9. Mechanism of oxytocin and vasopressin release by the posterior pituitary. The peptide hormones are synthe-sized by neurosecretory cells of the paraventricular and supraoptic nuclei in the hypothalamus, and transported in the form of secretory granules, down nerve axons in the pituitary stalk, to be stored in nerve terminals (close to blood capillaries) in the posterior pituitary lobe. Release occurs in response to suckling (oxytocin) or changes in blood volume/osmolarity (vasopressin).

the kidney, thereby reducing urine volume and conserving body fluid; AVP is therefore also referred to as the **anti-diuretic hormone (ADH)**. This effect is mediated by spe-cific AVP (V_2-type) receptors on the tubular cell surface, linked to a rise in intracellular cAMP. In *large quantities*, AVP has a direct vasoconstrictor action on blood vessels, and can increase the systemic blood pressure; the latter effect (mediated by AVP V_{1a}-type receptors, linked to IP_3 production) may be of significance in maintaining vas-cular tone in cases of severe haemorrhage: [selective V_{1a} receptor antagonists are currently being used to evaluate the possible pathophysiological role of AVP in the de-velopment of hypertension]. AVP can also facilitate the release of ACTH from the anterior pituitary in response to hypothalamic CRH (mediated via V_{1b} type receptors; see page 13).

Control of release of AVP is primarily influenced by:

1. *Plasma osmolarity* (mainly due to changes in plasma Na$^+$ level), sensed by specialized hypothalamic osmoreceptor

neurones connected with the SON. A relatively small increase in osmolarity (ca. 1–2%), increases the release of AVP so that less water is cleared and *vice versa**.

2. *Blood volume/arterial pressure:* sensory stimuli arising from systemic arterial, venous and atrial *baroreceptors* (stretch-sensitive) normally *inhibit* AVP secretion, via afferent autonomic nerve projections to the SON; a low plasma volume or pressure (more than 10–15% reduction, e.g. in response to haemorrhage) thus decreases baroreceptor stimulation resulting in an *increase* in circulating AVP.

An *increase* in AVP release also occurs in response to:

severe pain, fear, nausea, general anaesthesia or certain drugs/neurotransmitters e.g. nicotine, morphine (and other opiates), angiotensin II, prostaglandin E_2 and noradrenaline. Alcohol, however, *inhibits* AVP release (alcohol-induced diuresis).

☞ An increase in blood volume can also evoke the release of a 28 amino acid peptide from atrial muscle fibres, termed **atrial natriuretic peptide (ANP)** that causes an increase in the excretion of Na^+ and water by the kidneys (natriuresis) and vasodilatation. The heart itself can therefore behave as an important endocrine organ! Accordingly, ANP *inhibits* the secretion of AVP by the posterior pituitary, and may therefore contribute to the volume control of AVP release.

Hyposecretion of AVP, caused by damage or dysfunction (e.g. tumours) of the hypothalamus, can lead to *diabetes insipidus*, a condition in which excessively large amounts of dilute urine (10–15 litres/day) are produced by the kidneys. Patients experience frequent urination (*polyuria*) and excessive thirst and drinking (*polydipsia*).

Treatment. This involves the administration of synthetic **vasopressin** (*Pitressin*) by subcutaneous or intramuscular injection, or by intranasal administration of the vasopressin analogues **lypressin** (*Syntopressin*) or **desmopressin** (*Desmospray*) in the form of nasal spray solutions. Common side-effects associated with their use include nausea, nasal congestion and the desire to defaecate.

---

*Changes in blood volume and pressure can influence the threshold value (set-point) of the osmoreceptors to fluid osmolarity, so that a *fall* in volume/pressure *results in an enhancement* of osmoreceptor sensitivity and *vice versa*.

Hypersecretion of AVP: the rare condition of inappropriate AVP production is known as *Schwartz-Bartter syndrome* (or *SIADH: syndrome of inappropriate ADH*) in which excessive water retention (low serum osmolarity), a severe loss of plasma sodium (hyponatraemia), and a reduced ability to excrete diluted urine (high urine osmolarity) occur. Symptoms include weakness, lethargy, headache, weight gain, anorexia, and in extreme cases, confusion, seizures, and possible coma/death due to cerebral oedema; the excess AVP levels can arise from an ectopic AVP-secreting tumour (malignant bronchial neoplasm), certain pulmonary disorders (e.g. severe pneumonia, acute bronchitis), brain lesions affecting osmoreceptor function (minor head injury), or as a consequence of antidepressant/antipsychotic drug therapy (e.g. *fluoxetine, sertraline, imipramine, amitryptyline, haloperidol*).

Treatment. This involves prompt removal of the tumour where possible, or treatment of the underlying malignant disease; alternatively, water restriction, hypertonic (3%) saline infusion (together with a loop diuretic: frusemide) or oral administration of the AVP antagonist **demeclocycline** (*Ledermycin*) may be used.

Oxytocin

Although **oxytocin** has a similar structure to AVP, it has distinctly different physiological functions, mediated via specific oxytocin receptors on target cells (linked to IP_3 second messenger system). It is present in both sexes, but its effects are well understood only in females. Oxytocin stimulates the rhythmic contractions of uterine smooth muscle during parturition (childbirth), and also stimulates milk ejection from the lactating breast in response to infant suckling (milk *let-down*) by contracting the *myoepithelial cells* present in the alveolar secretory epithelium. Oxytocin contributes to, but is not essential for initiation or maintenance of labour.

Control of release: Activation of sensory nerve endings in the nipple during suckling, and the uterus during childbirth, ultimately stimulate release of oxytocin from the posterior pituitary; these reflexes (relayed to the hypothalamus via the spinothalamic tract) represent good examples of *neurogenic feedback* control mechanisms.

Disorders of oxytocin secretion are rarely encountered. Synthetic **oxytocin** (*Syntocinon*) is available for clinical use in the form of an injection, given by slow intravenous infusion for the induction of labour, where the uterine effort is inadequate, and also to stimulate uterine contractions after childbirth and delivery of the placenta, thereby lessening the danger of uterine haemorrhage. ∎

Review Questions

Question 1: State the location of the pituitary gland and outline its anatomical arrangement.

Question 2: List the main trophic hormones secreted by the anterior pituitary, describe their major target organ effects, and outline the mechanisms controlling their release.

Question 3: List the main hypothalamic releasing/inhibiting hormones and describe how they influence the anterior pituitary.

Question 4: Describe the effects of hypothalamic GnRH, CRH, TRH, dopamine, GHRH and somatostatin (SS).

Question 5: What is GnRH-associated peptide (GAP); how does it affect prolactin release?

Question 6: Describe (giving examples) the clinical uses of (a) GnRH analogues (b) octreotide (SS analogue).

Question 7: What is the significance of melanocyte stimulating hormone (MSH) in man? What is the structural relationship between MSH and corticotrophin (ACTH)?

Question 8: What type of drug is aminoglutethimide? Under what conditions may it be used therapeutically?

Question 9: Describe the consequences of excessive prolactin secretion and how this may be treated.

Question 10: Describe the consequences of under- or oversecretion of GH in early life and in adulthood. Give the appropriate treatments for each condition.

Question 11: List the major symptoms of acromegaly.

Question 12: What is the glucose suppression test? How may it be used in the diagnosis of GH hypersecretion?

Question 13: Explain briefly, the morphology of the posterior pituitary gland.

Question 14: Name the two hormones secreted by the posterior pituitary and state from which hypothalamic nuclei they originate.

Question 15: Describe the principal actions of vasopressin (AVP) and explain the mechanisms controlling its release. By what other name is this hormone usually referred to?

Question 16: What are the factors that control the release of atrial natriuretic peptide (ANP)? Describe the main effects of this peptide in the body.

Question 17: Describe the cause, symptoms and treatment of diabetes insipidus.

Question 18: What are the causes of Schwartz-Bartter syndrome (or SIADH: syndrome of inappropriate ADH)? Describe the main symptoms and treatment of this condition.

Question 19: Describe the main actions of oxytocin and explain the mechanisms controlling its release.

Question 20: Give the clinical uses for synthetic oxytocin.

Clinical Case Studies

Patient 1

A 17 year old girl was referred for evaluation of primary amenorrhoea. The patient was totally asymptomatic and denied use of the oral contraceptive pill or any other medications. She had no previous illnesses. A pregnancy test was negative. Clinical examination was normal. She had no galactorrhoea, and external genitalia were normal.

Laboratory investigation showed that her full blood count (FBC), urinalysis and serum electrolytes were normal. Blood chemistry, plasma cortisol and thyroid function tests were also normal. Her plasma oestradiol level was 50 pg/ml (normal >25 pg/ml), luteinizing hormone (LH) was 4.7 mU/ml (normal 4–30 mU/ml) and follicle stimulating hormone (FSH) was 5 mU/ml (normal 4–30 mU/ml). However, serum prolactin was elevated at 231 ng/ml (normal <20 ng/ml). An MRI (magnetic resonance image) of the head revealed a 6 mm pituitary microadenoma.

Question 1:   *What are the causes of hyperprolactinaemia?*
Question 2:   *What impact does hyperprolactinaemia have on reproductive functions?*
Question 3:   *What is the treatment for microprolactinoma?*

Answer 1:   *Hyperprolactinaemia* may result from physiological conditions (stress, pregnancy, infant suckling); pharmacological factors (drugs: dopamine receptor antagonists [e.g phenothiazines, butyrophenones, metoclopramide], reserpine or methyldopa [depletors of hypothalamic dopamine], oestrogens, opiates, monoamine oxidase (MAO) inhibitors, cimetidine, verapamil) or pathological factors (pituitary tumours, pituitary stalk lesion, primary hypothyroidism, chronic renal failure or severe liver disease).

Answer 2:   Hyperprolactinaemia decreases the activity of the hypothalamic GnRH pulse generator, leading to reduced gonadotrophin production/secretion and consequent low sex steroid levels. The LH/FSH and oestradiol levels were however, normal in this patient. Excess prolactin may also directly interfere with gonadotrophin action on the gonads, resulting in a functional hypogonadism; the outcome will be menstrual dysfunction (amenorrhoea) and infertility; (decreased libido, impotence and infertility in men). There is growing evidence that when hypogonadism develops, the risk of *osteopenia* (low bone mass) also increases.

Answer 3:   Treatment with a dopamine D_2 receptor agonist such as *bromocriptine* is the initial choice for management of microprolactinomas (tumours <10 mm in size). This agent mimics the normal inhibitory 'tone' exerted by hypothalamic dopamine-secreting neurones on pituitary prolactin secretion, and may reduce serum prolactin concentration and tumour size without the need for surgical removal; [bromocriptine can also be used to treat larger (>10 mm) prolactin-secreting tumours (macroprolactinomas) prior to surgery; these are often associated with severe visual field defects].

    The patient was started on *bromocriptine (2.5 mg daily, at bed time)* and the dose increased to 5 mg daily over a period of 6 weeks. By the 10th week, the prolactin level had been completely normalized (19 ng/ml), and the patient had her first menstrual period. An MRI of the head at 6 months, showed a normal pituitary gland. The patient is currently euprolactinaemic on a maintenance dose of bromocriptine (2.5 mg daily).

Patient 2

A 45 year old man presented at the emergency clinic complaining of increasing headache and double vision over the past two days. Past medical history included a ten year history of decreased sexual drive, impotence, tiredness, cold intolerance and arthritic pain in the hands and feet. He had also noticed that he shaved less frequently than before, his wedding ring no longer fitted him, and that his shoe size had progressively increased over the years. His facial features had also changed, particularly his nose and jaw. Clinical examination revealed a blood pressure of 105/65 mmHg (supine) with postural hypotension, lack of underarm and pubic hair, pale, dry, thickened skin, and prominent enlargement of the nose, lips tongue, ears and lower jaw. The hands and feet were also enlarged and 'doughy'. Deep tendon reflexes showed a delayed relaxation phase. A visual field test revealed a bitemporal hemianopia. The patient was admitted for further evaluation.

An MRI (magnetic resonance image) of the head showed an enlarged pituitary, with some suprasellar extension. Laboratory investigation indicated that FBC and blood chemistry were normal, although plasma glucose was 10 mmol/l (normal 3.6–6.4 mmol/l) and phosphate 5.1 mg/dl (normal 2.5–4.8 mg/dl). Serum electrolytes were: Na$^+$ 129 mmol/l (normal 135–145 mmol/l), K$^+$ 4.6 mmol/l (normal 3.5–5 mmol/l. Plasma cortisol at 8 a.m. was 4 μg/dl (normal 5–20 μg/dl), ACTH 20 pg/ml (normal 40–100 pg/ml), thyroxine (T$_4$) 1.8 μg/dl (normal 4–12 μg/dl), TSH <0.5 μU/ml (normal 0.5–5 μU/ml), LH 2 mU/ml (normal 4–30 mU/ml), testosterone 168 ng/dl (normal male 300–1110 ng/dl), GH 62 ng/ml (normal <5 ng/ml) and IGF-1 560 ng/ml (normal male adult 40–180 ng/ml). Serum prolactin was normal.

Question 1:   *What is this patient most likely suffering from? What is causing his chronic and acute symptoms?*

Question 2:   *What is the explanation of the laboratory findings?*

Question 3:   *How would this condition be treated?*

Answer 1:   This patient is showing classic signs of *chronic acromegaly with multiple endocrine deficits (hypopituitarism)* due to progressive growth of a pituitary tumour, secreting excess amounts of growth hormone (GH); [ectopic production of GHRH may also lead to pituitary GH oversecretion]. The patient also shows acute symptoms of optic compression (revealed by the visual field disturbances) that occurs when the pituitary tumour enlarges sufficiently to compress the central part of the optic chiasm. The main features of acromegaly include a gradual change in facial features (prominent brow, large nose, lips, tongue and protruding jaw) and overgrowth of the hands and feet, developing over a period of years; such patients can also show symptoms of glucose intolerance (diabetes), and arthritic pain in the extremities.

Answer 2:   The condition is characterized by an elevated plasma levels of GH and IGF-1 (insulin-like growth factor-1), although this in itself may not be diagnostic; both serum calcium and phosphate levels may also be increased in acromegalics. The associated hypopituitarism is caused through interruption of normal pituitary function by the expanding tumour; it is indicated by the low serum levels of testosterone, cortisol and thyroxine, with concomitant low levels of LH and ACTH and TSH. The resulting condition is a mixed clinical picture of hypogonadism (decreased libido and facial, axillary/pubic hair growth), hypothyroidism (dry, coarse skin, fatigue cold intolerance, delayed tendon reflexes) and hypoadrenalism (pale skin, mild hypotension).

Answer 3:   One day after admission, the patient's headache and visual disturbances became more acute, and a decision to remove the pituitary tumour by open transfrontal surgery was made, with abrupt improvement in visual field abnormalities the next day. The patient was then placed on oral replacement therapy (hydrocortisone, testosterone and thyroxine) to correct for endocrine deficiencies. The serum GH, and blood glucose/phosphate levels normalized after three days. Recession of soft tissue overgrowth was observed over several months, although there was no indication of a recovery of pituitary function. A repeat MRI scan one year post-operatively showed no recurrence of the tumour; the patient was maintained on replacement therapy.

Removal of pituitary tumours by trans-sphenoidal or open transfrontal surgery is used when the tumour size has expanded sufficiently to cause compression of the optic chiasm; with smaller tumours producing no pressure symptoms and not associated with significant hypopituitarism, the excess GH secretion (with some tumour shrinkage) can be achieved by administration of the dopamine receptor agonist *bromocriptine (10–20 mg daily)* or the long-acting somatostatin analogue *octreotide (0.1–0.2 mg, 3–4 times daily; subcutaneous)*.

UK/USA Drugs — Trade names		
	UK	**USA**
Hypothalamic hormones		
Gonadotrophin releasing hormone (GnRH)	Feritral	Factrel
		Lutrepulse
GnRH agonists	Buserelin	Supprelin
	Goserelin	Lupron
	Leuprorelin	Synarel
	Nafarelin	
Thyrotrophin releasing hormone (TRH)	Protirelin	Relefact TRH
GHRH analogue (Sermorelin)	Geref	
Somatostatin analogue (Octreotide)	Sandostatin	Sandostatin
Pituitary hormones		
Adrenocorticotrophic hormone (ACTH)		Acthar
ACTH analogue (Tetracosactrin)	Syncathen	Cortrosyn
Human growth hormone (GH)	Humatrope	Humatrope
		Protropin/Nutropin
Vasopressin (AVP)	Pitressin	Pitressin
Vasopressin analogues:		
Lypressin	Syntopressin	Diapid
Desmopressin	DDAVP	DDAVP*
	Desmospray	
Oxytocin	Syntocinon	Syntocinon
		Pitocin
Dopamine agonists		
Bromocriptine	Parlodel	Parlodel
Cabergoline	Dostinex	
Quinagolide	Norprolac	
Dopamine antagonists		
Haloperidol	Serenace	Haldol
Trifluoperazine	Stelazine	Stelazine

* DDAVP: 1-desamino-8-D-arginine vasopressin

References

Books

- **Ascoli M, Segaloff DL.** (1996). Adenohypophyseal hormones and their hypothalamic releasing factors. In *Goodman & Gilman's The Pharmacological Basis of Therapeutics*, edited by JG Hardman, LE Limbird, A Goodman, Gilman *et al.*, 9th ed. McGraw-Hill, USA, pp. 1363–1382
- **Carola R, Harley JP, Noback CR.** (1990). The endocrine system. In *Human Anatomy & Physiology*, McGraw-Hill, Inc, USA, pp. 474–504
- **Chandrasoma P, Taylor CR.** (1991). The pituitary gland. In *Concise Pathology*, 1st ed. Prentice-Hall, USA, pp. 833–838
- **Fitzgerald PA.** (1992). Pituitary disorders. In *Handbook of Clinical Endocrinology*, 2nd ed. Prentice-Hall, USA, pp. 1–72
- **Genuth SM.** (1993). The hypothalamus and pituitary gland. In *Physiology*, edited by RM Berne, MN Levy, 3rd ed. Mosby-Year Book Inc, USA, pp. 897–931
- **Goodman HM.** (1988). Pituitary gland. In *Basic Medical Endocrinology*, Raven Press, New York, pp. 27–44
- **Guyton AC, Hall JE.** (1996). The pituitary hormones and their control by the hypothalamus. In *Textbook of Medical Physiology*, 9th ed. WB Saunders Company, USA, pp. 933–944
- **Hassan T.** (1985). The pituitary gland. In *A Guide to Medical Endocrinology*, Macmillan Publishers Ltd, pp. 22–43
- **Hedge GA, Colby HD, Goodman RL.** (1987). The brain-pituitary interface. In *Clinical Endocrine Physiology*, WB Saunders Co, Philadelphia, Chapters 3–5, pp. 53–98
- **Junqueira LC, Carneiro J, Long JA.** (1986). Pituitary & Hypothalamus. In *Basic Histology*, 5th ed. Lange Medical Publications, Connecticut, pp. 435–445
- **McCann SM.** (1988). The anterior pituitary and hypothalamus. In *Textbook of Endocrine Physiology*, edited by JE Griffin, SR Ojeda. Oxford University Press, New York, pp. 70–99
- **Samson WK.** (1988). The posterior pituitary and water metabolism. In *Texbook of Endocrine Physiology*, edited by JE Griffin, SR Ojeda. Oxford University Press, New York, pp. 100–111
- **Thibodeau GA, Patton KT.** (1993). The endocrine system. In *Anatomy & Physiology*, 2nd ed. Mosby-Year Book Inc, USA, pp. 402–439
- **Tyrrell JB, Findling JW, Aron DC.** (1994). Hypothalamus and pituitary. In *Basic & Clinical Endocrinology*, edited by FS Greenspan, JD Baxter, 4th ed. Appleton & Lange, Connecticut, pp. 64–127

General

- **ABPI Data Sheet Compendium 1994–1995.** (1994). Datapharm Publications Ltd, London
- **British National Formulary.** (1996). Drugs used in the treatment of disorders of the endocrine system, British Medical Association and Royal Pharmaceutical Society of Great Britain, Chapter 6, pp. 285–327

- **Baird JD, Irvine WJ, Edwards CRW.** (1987). Endocrine and metabolic diseases. In *Davidson's Principles & Practice of Medicine*, edited by J Macleod, C Edwards, I Bouchier, 15th ed. Churchill Livingstone, pp. 423–492
- **Ellsworth AJ, Bray RF, Bray SB, Geyman JP.** (1991). *The Family Practice Drug Handbook*, Mosby-Year Book Inc, USA
- **Greenstein B.** (1994). *Endocrinology at a glance*, Blackwell Science, Oxford
- **Hillson RM.** (1994). The drug therapy of endocrine and metabolic disorders. In *Oxford Texbook of Clinical Pharmacology and Drug Therapy*, edited by DG Grahame-Smith, JK Aronson, 2nd ed. Oxford University Press, pp. 365–378
- **Kumar PJ, Clark ML.** (1990). Endocrinology. In *Clinical Medicine*, 2nd ed. Bailliere Tindall, pp. 764–831
- **Monthly Index of Medical Specialities (MIMS),** June 1997. Haymarket Medical Ltd, London
- **Plowman PN.** (1987). *Endocrinology and Metabolic Diseases*, John Wiley & Sons Ltd
- **Rang HP, Dale MM, Ritter JM.** (1995). The endocrine system. In *Pharmacology*, 3rd ed. Churchill Livingstone, pp. 417–426
- **Rees PJ, Williams DG.** (1995). Endocine disorders. In *Principles of Clinical Medicine*, Edward Arnold, pp. 517–554
- **Wilson JD, Foster DW.** (1992). *Williams Textbook of Endocrinology*, WB Saunders Co, Philadelphia

Journal Articles

- **Adams SP.** (1987). Structure and biologic properties of the atrial natriuretic peptides. *Endocrinol Metab Clin N Am*, 16, 1–17
- **Beckers A.** (1993). Presurgical octreotide treatment in acromegaly. *Acta Endocrinol*, 129, suppl. 1, 18–20
- **Chen C-LC.** (1993). Inhibin and activin as paracrine/autocrine factors. *Endocrinology*, 132, 4
- **Conn PM, Crowley WF Jr.** (1991). Gonadotrophin-releasing hormone and its analogues. *New Engl J Med*, 324, 93–103
- **Conn PM.** *et al.* (1986). Mechanism of action of gonadotrophin releasing hormone. *Annu Rev Physiol*, 48, 495–513
- **Frohman LA, Downs TR, Chomczynski P.** (1992). Regulation of growth hormone secretion. *Frontiers in Neuroendocrinology*, 13, 344–405
- **Gelato MC, Merriam GR.** (1986). Growth hormone releasing hormone. *Annu Rev Physiol*, 48, 569–591
- **Hsueh AJW,** *et al.* (1987). Heterodimers and homodimers of inhibin subunits have different paracrine action in the modulation of luteinizing hormone-stimulated androgen biosynthesis. *Proc Natl Acad Sci USA*, 84, 5082–5086
- **Jaffe CA, Barkan AL.** (1994). Acromegaly: recognition and treatment. *Drugs*, 47, 425–445

- **Laron Z.** (1993). Somatomedin-1 (insulin-like growth factor-I) in clinical use. *Drugs*, 45, 1–8
- **Laron Z.** (1995). Growth hormone secretagogues. *Drugs*, 50, 595–601
- **Marcus R,** *et al.* (1990). Effects of short term administration of recombinant human growth hormone to elderly people. *J Clin Endocrinol Metab*, 70, 519–527
- **Patel YC, Srikanat CB.** (1986). Somatostatin mediation of adenohypophysial secretion. *Annu Rev Physiol*, 48, 551–567
- **Rivier CL, Plotsky PM.** (1986). Mediation by corticotrophin releasing factor (CRF) of adenohypophysial hormone secretion. *Annu Rev Physiol*, 48, 475–494
- **Rivier JP,** *et al.* (1992). GnRH antagonists: a synopsis. *Contraception*, 46, 109–112
- **Ruberg M,** *et al.* (1987). Stimulation of prolactin release by vasoactive intestinal peptide (VIP). *Eur J Pharmacol*, 51, 319–320.
- **Rudman D,** *et al.* (1990). Effects of human growth hormone in men over 60 years old. *New Engl J Med*, 323, 1–6
- **Strobl JS, Thomas MJ.** (1994). Human growth hormone. *Pharmacol Rev*, 46, 1–34
- **Wintzen M, Gilchrest BA.** (1996). Proopiomelanocortin, its derived peptides, and the skin. *J Invest Dermatol*, 106, 3–10
- **Woodruff TK, Mayo KE.** (1990). Regulation of inhibin synthesis in the rat ovary. *Annu Rev Physiol*, 52, 807–821
- **Zeidel ML.** (1990). Renal actions of atrial natriuretic peptide: regulation of collecting duct sodium and water transport. *Annu Rev Physiol*, 52, 747–759

3 The Adrenal Gland

Structure and Histology

The adrenal glands are situated above the upper pole of each kidney, embedded in fatty tissue, and receive a copious arterial blood supply from the aorta and renal arteries. Each gland (weighing 6–10 g) consists of an *outer cortex* and an *inner medulla* which secrete quite different types of hormones (*steroids* and *catecholamines* respectively). An extensive sympathetic (preganglionic) nerve supply runs to the *medulla*, which secretes **adrenaline (80%)** and **noradrenaline (20%)**. Unlike the latter, the adrenal *cortex* is essential to life, and consists of three separate epithelial cell layers arranged into three zones (Figure 3.1):

The outer layer: (*zona glomerulosa*): secretes **mineralocorticoids**; involved in Na^+/H_2O balance

The middle layer: (*zona fasciculata*): secretes **glucocorticoids**: involved in regulating protein/carbohydrate metabolism; also secretes some **sex steroids**

The inner layer: (*zona reticularis*): secretes **glucocorticoids** and some **sex steroids**

☞ The adrenal secretion of sex steroids (**testosterone, dehydroepiandrosterone, oestradiol,** and **progesterone**) is normally small and physiologically insignificant, compared with the testicular and ovarian secretion of these hormones (see Chapter 6). In females, the growth of underarm (axillary) and pubic hair is dependent on adrenal androgen secretion.

Histology

The *zona glomerulosa* forms a very narrow zone immediately beneath the thick outer connective tissue capsule that surrounds the gland. The cells are small, ovoid in shape and arranged into small ovoid clusters or 'arches': these cells produce the mineralocorticoid hormone **aldosterone**, involved in regulating Na^+, K^+ and water balance in the body.

The *zona fasciculata* is the widest of the three cortical zones, and consists of larger cells arranged radially into

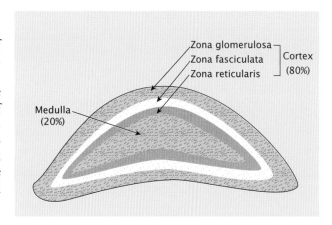

Figure 3.1. Schematic cross-section of an adrenal gland, showing the different functional zones. The cortex and medulla are functionally distinct types of endocrine tissue.

long columns, with blood capillaries running in between. The cytoplasm of the cells contains numerous lipid droplets, which represent a precursor store for the synthesis of **glucocorticoid** steroids: these are important in maintaining life and regulating protein and carbohydrate metabolism.

The innermost *zona reticularis* is composed of irregular columns of smaller epithelial cells with capillary spaces in between. The cells are smaller and contain fewer lipid droplets.

The *adrenal medulla* (derived embryologically from neural crest tissue) consists of clusters of large roundish *chromaffin cells* which produce *catecholamines*, surrounded by a network of reticular fibres, blood vessels and autonomic nerve fibres; the cells are of two types, storing either **adrenaline** or **noradrenaline**, and may be considered as modified sympathetic ganglion cells (devoid of axons and dendrites). Indeed, small numbers of sympathetic ganglionic neurones, occurring singly or in small groups, may also be found within the medullary tissue. Chromaffin cells are so called because they exhibit numerous brown *chromaffin granules* (100–300 nm diameter) when stained with chromium salts (*chromaffin reaction*). Secretion of catecholamines into the bloodstream occurs in direct response to stimulation of preganglionic (cholinergic) sympathetic nerve

25

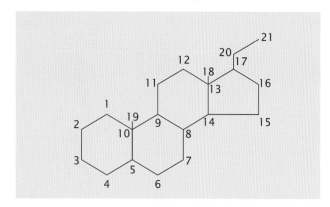

Figure 3.2. The basic C_{17} cyclopentanoperhydrophenanthrene steroid nucleus, with numbers indicating the position of carbon atoms and possible side chains.

fibres as part of the so-called "fight-or-flight" response to stress.

Biosynthesis and Release of Adrenocortical Hormones

All the adrenalcortical hormones are polycyclic *steroids*, derived initially from *plasma cholesterol*, and bear the same basic 17-carbon steroid *cyclopentanoperhydrophenanthrene* nucleus (Figure 3.2). Some cholesterol is also formed intrinsically from acetate and acetylcoenzyme A. The initial biosynthetic steps occurring within the adrenal cells are common; however, the hormone end-products may vary according to the type of carbon side chain or groupings attached at position C_{17}.

Generally,

C_{21} compounds can possess either glucocorticoid, mineralo-corticoid, or progestogenic activity;

C_{19} compounds usually possess androgenic (masculinizing) activity, whereas,

C_{18} compounds can have oestrogenic (feminizing) activity.

A double bond between C_4–C_5 (written as Δ^5) and a ketone group at C_3 appear to be essential for normal adrenocorticoid activity; potent *glucocorticoids* generally also require hydroxyl groups at positions 11 and 21, whereas active *mineralocorticoids* require an aldehyde group at position 18 (Figure 3.3.).

☞ Steroid hormones are not 'flat' molecules, but have a complex three-dimensional shape.

Control of Release

Adrenal steroids are not stored within the adrenocortical cells in significant amounts, but are liberated as soon as they are synthesized. The rate of glucocorticoid synthesis and secretion (principally **cortisol**) is controlled exclusively by the anterior pituitary hormone **corticotrophin (ACTH)** under negative feedback control (see Chapter 1). The effects of ACTH on the adrenal cells are believed to be mediated by specific membrane receptors linked to intracellular cyclic AMP production. ACTH is also necessary for the normal growth and maintenance of the adrenal cortex (trophic effect), which may undergo atrophy (gradual wasting away) after surgical removal of the pituitary. Cortisol secretion, like that of ACTH shows a circadian rhythm (24 hour periodicity), with the highest blood levels being exhibited in the morning, before waking; the physiological significance of this variation however, remains uncertain.

By contrast, the regulation of mineralocorticoid (mainly **aldosterone**) secretion, is largely mediated by the **renin-angiotensin system** involving the kidney (see p. 34). Both glucocorticoids and mineralocorticoids are bound to plasma proteins in the circulation (mainly **transcortin** — an α_2-globulin, and albumin) leaving only about 10% free and metabolically active; aldosterone also has a specific binding globulin, although its degree of binding to protein is relatively less. The free plasma cortisol concentration (about 100–700 nmol/l at 9.00 a.m.) is about 2000 times greater than the plasma aldosterone concentration (50–300 pmol/l).

Glucocorticoids

Cortisol (also known as *hydrocortisone*) is the principal glucocorticoid secreted in man, although some **corticosterone** is also produced.

The main actions of the glucocorticoids are:

1. Control of carbohydrate, protein and fat metabolism.
2. Suppression of tissue inflammation in response to injury.
3. Suppression of immune response to foreign antigens.
4. Increase in capacity of the body to withstand various noxious stimuli (stresses).

☞ The anti-inflammatory and immunosuppressant actions only become apparent at high or therapeutic concentrations of glucocorticoids.

Carbohydrate Metabolism

Cortisol increases blood glucose levels by stimulating glucose formation in the liver (*gluconeogenesis*) from circulating amino acid precursors, and promotes the storage of liver

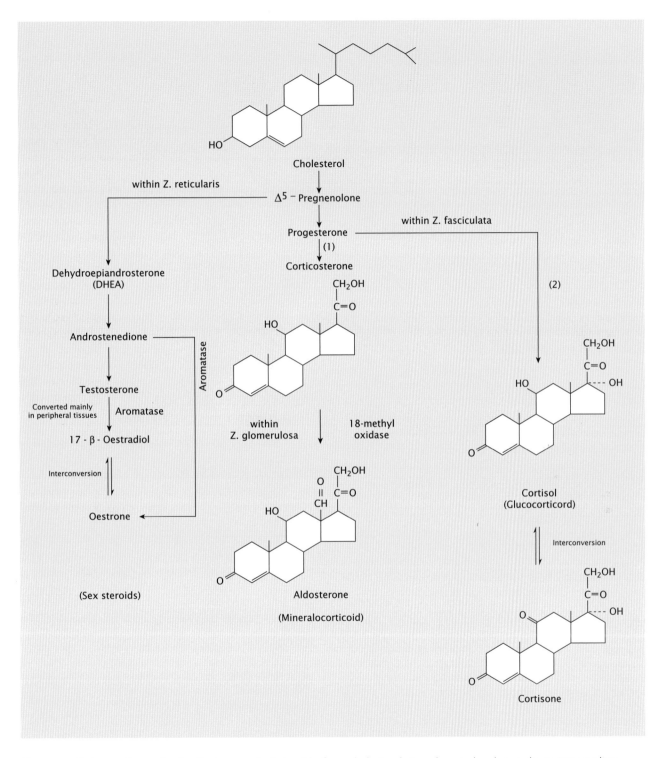

Figure 3.3. Pathways for synthesis of adrenocortical steroids from cholesterol: (numbers in brackets indicate intermediate synthesis steps omitted for clarity). Note that the conversion of corticosterone to aldosterone occurs only within the *zona glomerulosa* which lacks *17α-hydroxylase* enzyme activity, and is thus unable to produce cortisol or androgens; also the enzyme *aromatase* (oestrogen synthetase) catalyses the conversion of testosterone to oestradiol, as well as the direct conversion of androstenedione to oestrone.

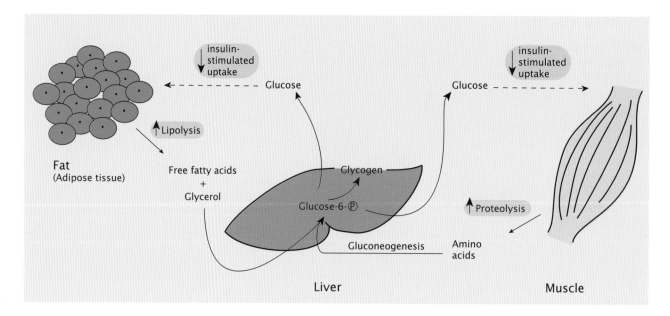

Figure 3.4. Principal metabolic actions of cortisol. Protein and fat breakdown are promoted with a resultant release of amino acids and glycerol substrates, utilized by the liver for glucose and glycogen synthesis. The insulin-sensitive uptake of glucose by fat and muscle cells is also inhibited.

glycogen; the effects are accomplished by the induced production of additional metabolic enzymes involved in gluconeogenesis and glycogen synthesis. Cortisol also *antagonizes* the action of **insulin** on glucose uptake into muscle and adipose tissue; a prolonged action of cortisol may therefore lead to a high blood sugar level (*hyperglycaemia*).

Protein Metabolism

Cortisol inhibits amino acid uptake and protein synthesis in peripheral tissues. It also promotes protein breakdown in muscle, skin and bone, with consequent release of amino acids into the blood (utilized for gluconeogenesis). The synthesis of glucose thus occurs at the expense of protein catabolism. Excess cortisol can therefore lead to muscle wasting as well as loss of protein (collagen) from the skin and capillary walls (increased tendency to bruise) and bone matrix.

Fat (Lipid) Metabolism

Cortisol stimulates fat breakdown (lipolysis) in adipose tissue, with release of fatty acids and glycerol (for gluconeogenesis), while inhibiting fat synthesis. Excess cortisol may cause *an unusual redistribution of body fat* with increased deposition in the face and trunk, and between the shoulders (symptoms of *Cushing's syndrome;* see below). The principal metabolic actions of the glucocorticoids are summarized in Figure 3.4.

Anti-Inflammatory and Immunosuppressive Actions

Cortisol (and other glucocorticoids) when administered at relatively high pharmacologic doses, inhibit the normal inflammatory process which occurs when tissue is damaged. This action underlies the therapeutic use of corticosteroids in the treatment of certain severe chronic inflammatory conditions e.g. rheumatic diseases (rheumatic fever, rheumatoid arthritis), allergic rhinitis and eczematous skin disorders. A wide range of synthetic glucocorticoids are now available for systemic and topical use.

Some commonly used glucocorticoid preparations include:

1. **Prednisolone**   (*Prednesol, Deltastab, Precortisyl*)
2. **Betamethasone**   (*Betnelan, Betnovate [as valerate]*)
3. **Dexamethasone**   (*Decadron*)
4. **Triamcinolone**   (*Adcortyl*)
5. **Beclomethasone**   (*Propaderm*)
6. **Fluocinolone**   (*Synalar*)

☞ The introduction of a 9α-fluoro group into the steroid ring (as in *betamethasone, dexamethasone* or *triamcinolone*) greatly enhances the anti-inflammatory activity of the molecule, as does the substitution of a valerate group at position C_{17}, or the insertion of a double bond between C_1 and C_2 (as in *prednisolone*).

ANTI-INFLAMMATORY EFFECT

The mechanisms underlying the anti-inflammatory actions of glucocorticoids are varied and complex, as are the sequence of reactions involved in the inflammatory response itself. The latter may be regarded as a primary defensive reaction of tissues to trauma, harmful invading organisms or chemical substances and other antigenic agents, and is intended to protect the host tissue from further damage.

Inflammation is characterized by a reddening, warmth, swelling and pain at the site of injury, reflecting a localized vasodilatation, leak of protein and fluid from microcapillaries and venules, and release of chemical pain mediators; the increased blood flow facilitates the delivery of phagocytic leucocytes (e.g. neutrophils) and serum factors to the injured area. These defensive processes are initiated primarily by the production of **prostaglandins, thromboxanes, platelet activating factor (PAF)** and **leukotrienes** derived from the metabolism of the fatty acid **arachidonic acid.**

Glucocorticoids are known to inhibit the synthesis and release of these important inflammatory mediators by suppressing the activity of the enzyme *phospholipase A$_2$ (PLA$_2$)*, involved in the formation of arachidonic acid from cell membrane phospholipid (*phosphatidyl choline*). This effect is mediated indirectly via the induction of a phosphoprotein *lipocortin-1*, that inhibits PLA$_2$ activity, and also directly by inhibition of inducible PLA$_2$ synthesis. Inhibition of the production of *cyclo-oxygenase-2 (COX-2)*, an inducible form of the enzyme responsible for conversion of arachidonic acid to pro-inflammatory-prostaglandins has also been recently demonstrated.

Other factors that contribute towards the anti-inflammatory effect include:

1. Stabilization of intracellular lysosomal membranes, thereby preventing release of proteolytic lysosomal enzymes in inflamed tissue.
2. Decrease in recruitment and phagocytic activity of blood leucocytes at specific sites of tissue inflammation, [due to decreased release of chemoattractants and endothelial cell activators].
3. Decrease in the proliferation and deposition of collagen fibrils by fibroblasts at the site of injury.
4. Decrease in the synthesis of a number of epithelial cell-derived peptide mediators (*cytokines*) e.g. *GM-CSF (granulocyte macrophage colony stimulating factor), tumour necrosis factor-α (TNF-α)* and *interleukins-1, 6 and 8 (IL-1, IL-6, IL-8)*, involved in the initiation and enhancement of inflammation.

☞ Cyclo-oxygenase (COX) is known to exist in at least two distinct isoforms, COX-1 and COX-2. COX-1 is expressed in most tissues and has important physiological functions including provision of small amounts of prostaglandins necessary for gastroprotection, platelet aggregation and the control of renal blood flow, whereas COX-2 is only present at low levels in normal tissue, but is induced locally by proinflammatory stimuli (e.g. cytokines, growth factors, bacterial endotoxins). Corticosteroids preferentially inhibit the activity of COX-2 (and subsequent prostaglandin production), thereby producing a potent anti-inflammatory effect.

The recently developed nonsteroidal anti-inflammatory drug (NSAID) meloxicam (Mobic) also shows selective effects towards COX-2 and is intended for treatment of rheumatoid arthritis and other inflammatory conditions, while minimizing the risk of gastric or renal side effects (resulting from COX-1 inhibition).

In large doses, glucocorticoids can also have *anti-allergic* effects due partly, to an inhibition of mast cell development and migration, and the formation and release of histamine from mast cell granules. This property, although delayed in onset, can be useful in the adjunctive treatment (along with adrenaline) of emergency cases of severe asthma and anaphylactic shock. In these cases, **hydrocortisone** (*Hydrocortistab*) would be given by slow intravenous injection.

IMMUNOSUPPRESSIVE EFFECT

Therapeutic doses of glucocorticoids have major effects on the circulating cells (lymphocytes) involved in the immune response; principally, they inhibit the synthesis and action of essential peptide factors required for triggering the proliferation and maturation of T-lymphocyte cells (thymus-derived) within lymphoid tissue, following antigen presentation. These factors include **interleukin-1 (IL-1)**, **interleukin-6 (IL-6)** and **tumour necrosis factor-α (TNF-α)** (*cytokines* released from antigen-presenting macrophages) and **interleukin-2 (IL-2)** (a *lymphokine* released from T-cells). This ultimately leads to a reduced number of circulating T-cells, and also B-lymphocytes (bone-marrow derived) therefore resulting in a decreased antibody production (immunosuppression). A direct inhibition of antibody formation and a killing of B- and T-cells may occur at high glucocorticoid concentrations; a reduction in size of the thymus gland (and other lymphoid tissue) can also result following sustained high therapeutic doses.

Glucocorticoids also interfere with the interaction of other important lymphokine mediators (produced by T-lymphocytes) with their target cells (e.g. *macrophage activation and migration factors, B-cell helper factors* and immune *interferon-γ*, an important anti-viral molecule).

The immunosuppressive action of glucocorticoids can be useful therapeutically:

1. For the treatment of various autoimmune diseases;
2. In the prevention of tissue rejection following transplant or graft operations; however, since the resistance to infection will also be reduced, *antibiotics* must also be given concurrently.

Response to Stress

Unfavourable stresses such as *acute trauma, major surgery, severe infection, pain, haemorrhage, hypoglycaemia, cold, fever* or *emotional stimuli* can (via the release of negative feedback inhibition of the hypothalamic-pituitary axis; see Chapter 2) dramatically increase plasma cortisol levels, which appears to 'protect' the body against these stressful circumstances. In *adrenalectomized* patients, even relatively mild stress can prove fatal, unless replacement glucocorticoids are given. Apart from increasing blood levels of glucose and free fatty acids for energy sources, the nature of this protective action of cortisol towards stress is still largely unclear. Recent evidence however suggests that the pronounced inhibition of production of cytokines and other inflammatory/immune mediators by glucocorticoids, may be an important component of the 'stress protection' response, by preventing stress-induced defence reactions from 'overshooting' and becoming potentially damaging to the host. Accordingly, peripherally-produced cytokines like IL-1, IL-6 and TNF-α have been shown to directly stimulate release of CRH and ACTH from the hypothalamic-pituitary axis during inflammatory/immune stress, indicating an important regulatory link between the immune and central nervous systems under such conditions.

☞ Abrupt stopping of prolonged glucocorticoid therapy may (due to negative feedback effects on the anterior pituitary and hypothalamus; Chapter 1) result in adrenal insufficiency, and therefore an inability to withstand stressful stimuli. A gradual reduction of dosage over a period of weeks or months is therefore advisable, along with the carrying of *steroid treatment cards* to warn patients of possible complications.

Mechanism of Action

Cortisol permeates readily through target cell membranes and interacts with the C-terminal portion of a specific *glucocorticoid receptor protein (GR)* present predominantly in the cytosol. A change in conformation in the middle (DNA-binding) domain of the protein then allows it translocate into the nucleus and to bind reversibly with specific regulatory sites *(glucocorticoid response elements; GREs)* on target DNA molecules (close to promoter region of target genes), with a resultant induction or repression of gene transcription (Figure 3.5). Dimerization of the hormone-receptor complex is apparently necessary for correct interaction with the regulatory elements.

In the absence of glucocorticoid, inactive GR is associated with a blocking protein (*Hsp-90*, a so-called *heat shock protein*), that may also be important for maintaining the normal steroid binding activity of the receptor. The ability of the hormone to affect target cells is thus dependent on the presence of GR and its degree of inhibition by blocking proteins. In view of the complex intracellular mechanism of action of cortisol, its pharmacological effects may not be evident for hours or even days. A similar basic mode of action also applies to other steroid and thyroid hormones, for vitamin D and for retinoic acid (vitamin A acid); the GR protein is thus one member of a general steroid/thyroid hormone receptor superfamily.

Recent biochemical observations indicate that the GR (like other steroid hormone receptors) is in a partially phosphorylated state in the absence of ligand, and becomes *hyper*phosphorylated (by intracellular *kinases*) in the presence of hormone; this induced change is now regarded as an important step governing the subsequent transcriptional activity of the receptor.

☞ A decrease in the activity of the gene-transcription factor *AP-1 (activator protein-1)*, activated during chronic inflammation has been proposed to be an important mechanism underlying the anti-inflammatory and immunosuppressive action of glucocorticoids; the activated glucocorticoid receptor forms a protein-protein complex with AP-1 within the nucleus, thereby counteracting the activating effects of AP-1 on gene transcription.

Clinical Disorders

Hyposecretion of Glucocorticoids

Adrenalcortical insufficiency (*hypoadrenalism*), although rather uncommon, may either be *primary*, due to autoimmune adrenal disease affecting both adrenal cortices (*Addison's disease*) or *secondary* due to low ACTH levels (e.g. due to negative feedback on the hypothalamic-pituitary axis during prolonged corticosteroid therapy, or due to hypofunction of the pituitary *per se*). In the *former*, there is a deficiency in both *cortisol and aldosterone* production (see below).

Primary adrenal insufficiency may also arise as a consequence of metastatic infiltration, granulomatous disease involving the adrenal gland (tuberculosis, histoplasmosis, sarcoidosis), acute adrenal haemorrhage caused by meningococcal septicaemia or anticoagulant drug therapy, adrenalitis occurring in acquired immune deficiency syndrome (AIDS), or a congenital unresponsiveness to ACTH.

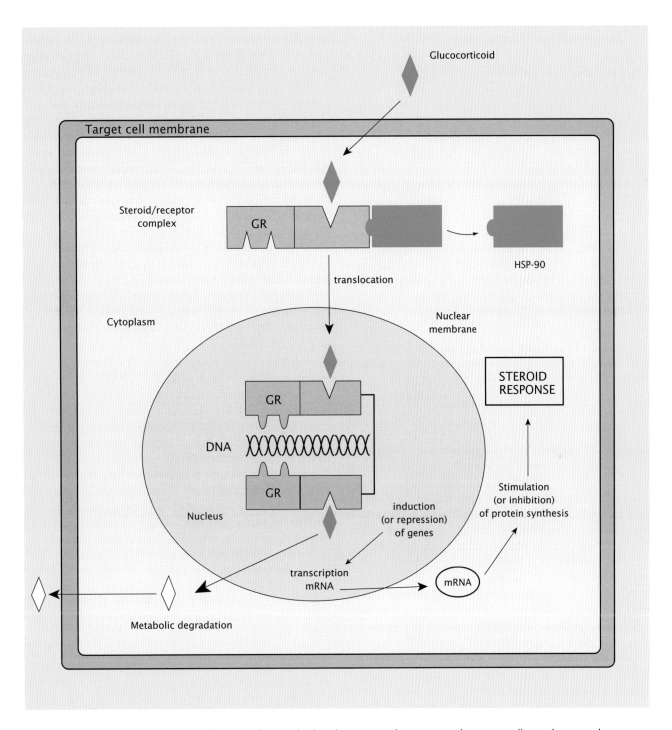

Figure 3.5. Intracellular mechanism of action of cortisol. The glucocorticoid penetrates the target cell membrane and combines with a specific glucocorticoid receptor (GR) present in the cytoplasm, to form a steroid/receptor complex. The interaction induces a conformational change in the receptor and dissociation of an associated heat shock protein (Hsp-90) before translocation into the nucleus to combine with target sites (glucocorticoid response elements) on DNA molecules, in a dimeric form. The induction (or repression) of target genes leads to stimulation (or inhibition) in synthesis of specific proteins that mediate the 'steroid response'.

☞ A rare defect in the adrenal ACTH receptor protein has been suggested as one possible cause of *familial glucocorticoid deficiency (FGD)*, an inherited syndrome characterized by an insensitivity of the adrenal gland to ACTH.

Clinical features of *Addison's disease* include:

1. *Muscle weakness*, postural hypotension and dehydration (due to aldosterone deficiency); salt craving; hypoglycaemia.
2. *Anorexia* and decrease in body weight.
3. *Nausea*, vomiting, diarrhoea; fever; abdominal pain.
4. *Tiredness* and *malaise*.
5. Low *levels of plasma cortisol*, associated with high *levels of ACTH*. Adrenal autoantibodies may also be present in the serum.
6. *Increased skin pigmentation* (lack of cortisol leads to an *increase* in plasma ACTH levels due to release from negative feedback; note that ACTH has MSH-like activity: see p. 11); the pigmentation is particularly prominent around scars, skin creases, elbows, knees and buttocks, the nipple area and the gums.

☞ *Low* plasma cortisol levels with *low* levels of ACTH would be expected in patients with *secondary hypoadrenalism*; low cortisol/high ACTH levels are also seen in cases of *congenital adrenal hyperplasia*, where enzyme defects occur in cortisol biosynthesis (see below).

Treatment. In patients with chronic adrenal insufficiency, combination replacement therapy with both glucocorticoid and mineralocorticoid compounds is necessary. A combination of **hydrocortisone** and **fludrocortisone** (a synthetic mineralocorticoid: *Florinef*) administered by mouth, is nowadays recommended. Alternatively, **cortisone acetate** (*Cortisyl*), which possesses virtually equal glucocorticoid and mineralocorticoid activity, may be used. Acute cases of adrenal insufficiency (*adrenal crisis*), as may occur in Addison's disease patients subjected to excessive stress, require an immediate intravenous infusion of **hydrocortisone** together with saline, to correct for low blood volume.

☞ In the *short ACTH stimulation test* of adrenocortical insufficiency, plasma cortisol levels are measured at 30 and 60 min following administration of a synthetic ACTH analogue (**tetracosactrin**; *Synacthen*; p. 11) by intramuscular or intravenous injection. In patients with primary adrenocortical failure, the expected rise in plasma cortisol level is not observed; (normally, a peak cortisol level of ≥18 μg/dl would be expected following administration of 250 μg tetracosactrin).

In *congenital (virilizing) adrenal hyperplasia*, there are inherited enzymatic defects in cortisol biosynthesis; any of the steroidogenic enzymes may be affected. Deficiency of *21β-hydroxylase*, one of the key enzymes in the cortisol (and aldosterone) synthetic pathway, leads to a reduction in cortisol secretion (with a compensatory rise in plasma ACTH) and a build up of adrenal androgenic steroid precursors (*17-hydroxy-progesterone, androstenedione* and ultimately *testosterone*; see Chapter 6). Aldosterone synthesis may also, occasionally be affected. The excess production of ACTH leads to an excessive growth (*hyperplasia*) of the adrenal cortex.

Apart from general symptoms of glucocorticoid/mineralocorticoid deficiency, female infants may show symptoms of masculinization at birth (abnormal sexual organs, clitoral enlargement) or later in life (precocious puberty, acne, hirsutism or amenorrhoea in adulthood). Affected male infants may go undetected at birth, unless significant salt-loss or shock under stress occurs.

Treatment involves carefully-dosed glucocorticoid (and if necessary, mineralocorticoid) replacement therapy to suppress excess ACTH (and therefore inappropriate steroid) secretion.

Hypersecretion of Glucocorticoids

Excess production of cortisol may result *either* from overproduction of ACTH (due to pituitary disease: 80% of cases, or by an ectopic ACTH-secreting tumour) *or* from an ACTH-independent adrenal cortical tumour (adenoma, micro- or macronodular adrenal hyperplasia or carcinoma). The majority of ectopic tumours secreting high levels of ACTH are thoracic in origin (bronchial, thymic, pancreatic or medullary thyroid tumours), some of which may be difficult to locate ('occult') using conventional X-ray or other modern radiographic imaging methods. In rare cases, an ectopic CRH-secreting tumour may be present.

The resultant condition of *hypercortisolism* (more prevalent in women) is called *Cushing's syndrome*. Its symptoms may also be induced after long-term therapy with glucocorticoids (e.g. for asthma, rheumatoid arthritis or inflammatory bowel disease).

☞ The condition of excess *pituitary* ACTH secretion is traditionally referred to as *Cushing's disease*.

The classical features of *Cushing's syndrome* are:

1. *Muscle weakness* and *wasting*; thin arms and legs — due to increased protein breakdown.
2. *Back pain* (due to *osteoporosis*); osteoporotic fractures of the hip, ribs or vertebrae may occur in the elderly.

☞ Excess cortisol (or glucocorticoid treatment) interferes with bone metabolism primarily by reducing the absorption of Ca^{2+} from the gastrointestinal tract (due to reduced formation of an active vitamin D metabolite; see Chapter 7), increasing renal Ca^{2+} excretion, inhibiting bone cell (osteoblast) function and also by enhancing (indirectly) the rate of bone resorption. Inhibition of protein synthesis leads to loss of vital collagen from the bone matrix.

3. *Tendency to bruise easily*, and development of *purple striae* within the skin (particularly on the thighs and abdomen) — due to defective protein synthesis.
4. *Redistribution of body fat tissue*, so that patient develops a *rounded (moon) face*, prominent abdomen (trunk obesity), *'buffalo' hump* and thin legs; the reasons for this fat redistribution remain uncertain.
5. *Virilization of females* (hair growth on face/body, amenorrhoea, acne) due to synthesis of abnormally high levels of *adrenal androgens*. The androgen precursors *dehydroepiandrosterone (DHEA)*, *DHEA sulphate (DHEAS)* and androstenedione are subsequently converted to *testosterone* in peripheral tissues.

☞ A similar excess in adrenal androgen production can occur in the condition of *congenital adrenal hyperplasia* (see above).

6. *Hyperglycaemia, polyuria* (excessive urination), *polydipsia* (excessive thirst), tendency towards *diabetes mellitus* (see Chapter 5).
7. *Psychological disturbances*, particularly in patients with a previous history of mental disorder; excess cortisol can lead to euphoria, hallucinations, paranoia or suicidal depression. The threshold for inducing seizure activity may also be reduced.
8. *High* levels of *plasma and urinary free cortisol* (with loss of diurnal variation), and *low (or undetectable)* levels of *plasma ACTH* (due to negative feedback inhibition by cortisol).

Treatment. This is usually by removal of the pituitary, ectopic (usually in lung) or adrenal tumour if possible, coupled with corticosteroid replacement therapy. When tumours are not easily located or inoperable, patients may undergo therapy with the steroid synthesis inhibitor **aminoglutethimide** (*Orimeten*; 250 mg–1 g daily; see also Chapter 6) together with supplementary corticosteroids if necessary. Dizziness, nausea, severe drowsiness and skin rashes may however occur as side effects of aminoglutethimide therapy.

Prolonged therapeutic use of synthetic glucocorticoids for their anti-inflammatory or immunosuppressive properties may also induce symptoms of Cushing's syndrome as detailed above; their gradual discontinuation should, however, lead to a resolution of the Cushingoid symptoms.

Metyrapone (*Metopirone*) is a competitive inhibitor of the 11β-hydroxylase enzyme involved in the final step of cortisol synthesis in the adrenal cortex; this drug may also be used in the treatment of Cushing's syndrome arising from an ectopic ACTH-secreting tumour (bronchial carcinoma), and also for controlling symptoms in patients prior to pituitary or adrenal surgery.

☞ In the *overnight dexamethasone suppression test* of suspected Cushing's syndrome, a patient is given a single 1 mg dose of **dexamethasone** at midnight, and the plasma cortisol level measured the next morning (8 a.m.). In a normal individual, the plasma cortisol would be reduced to a low level (<5 μg/dl), due to the negative feedback effects of dexamethasone; however, in a Cushing's syndrome patient, where the hypothalamic-pituitary axis would be under continual feedback suppression from cortisol, no lowering of the plasma cortisol level would be observed. Such patients would also fail to show the normal circadian rhythm of glucocorticoid secretion.

The overnight dexamethasone test would confirm the presence or absence of Cushing's syndrome but not readily distinguish between pituitary-dependent Cushing's syndrome and hypercortisolism due to ectopic ACTH secretion. In alternative *low and high dose dexamethasone suppression tests*, a 0.5 mg dose of dexamethasone is given initially every six hours for two days, followed by a 2 mg dose six hourly for another two days; plasma cortisol levels are measured at 8 am on days zero and two. Following the low dose test, a failure to suppress the excess cortisol production would confirm the presence of Cushing's syndrome; after the high dose test however, suppression of cortisol levels would be expected if the condition is pituitary-dependent (Cushing's *disease*), but not if it arises from ectopic ACTH/CRH secretion or an adrenal tumour.

In the *CRH stimulation test*, synthetic ovine CRH (oCRH) is given by intravenous bolus (1 μg/kg body weight), and plasma ACTH levels measured at regular intervals thereafter. In patients with pituitary Cushing's disease, a significant rise in ACTH would be expected, whereas patients with ectopic ACTH production would not generally show such a response.

Mineralocorticoids

Aldosterone is the principal potent mineralocorticoid secreted in man, although some **deoxycorticosterone** is also produced. Many other steroids can exert a similar (usually weaker) mineralo-corticoid action. Mineralocorticoids can also possess some glucocorticoid activity (and *vice versa*). Aldosterone is a very powerful mineralocorticoid, the active free concentration in the plasma being in the order of 100 pmol/l.

The main actions of aldosterone are:

1. Conservation of body sodium and excretion of potassium; aldosterone *increases* Na^+ reabsorption while promoting excretion of K^+ and H^+ across epithelial cell walls in the distal convoluted tubule and collecting ducts of the kidney. The resultant decrease in water excretion (by passive tubular reabsorption), increases blood volume.

2. Decrease in the ratio of sodium to potassium ion concentrations in sweat and in saliva; the increased inward transport of Na^+ (with passive efflux of K^+) occurs across the epithelial cell membranes of sweat and salivary gland ducts. In a hot climate, where excessive sweating may occur, the action of aldosterone would be important in preventing excessive Na^+ loss via this route.

3. Increase in the reabsorption of Na^+ from the colon, and increased excretion of K^+ in the faeces.

☞ Although only about 2% of the Na^+ filtered by the kidney is reabsorbed under the control of aldosterone, inhibitors of aldosterone action e.g. **spironolactone** (*Aldactone*) or **potassium canrenoate** (*Spiroctan-M*) will act as powerful *diuretics*, useful in the treatment of oedema. These drugs competitively antagonize the action of aldosterone on kidney tubule Na^+ reabsorption, so that more water is excreted in the urine.

Mechanism of Action

The effects of aldosterone on epithelial Na^+ reabsorption have a delayed (1–2 hour) onset, and are mediated intracellularly by interaction with a high affinity cytosolic (type I) mineralocorticoid receptor (highly homologous with the glucocorticoid receptor) which then binds with regulatory elements of nuclear DNA to induce the synthesis of a Na^+ transport protein (channel) (c.f. the genomic action of glucocorticoids; Figure 3.5). An increased synthesis of Na^+/K^+-ATPase molecules that pump Na^+ out of the tubular cells into the interstitial fluid, may also be initiated. The mechanisms underlying the K^+ and H^+ excretion effects however, are less well understood: the movement of K^+ into the tubular fluid is most likely a passive response to the increased intracellular Na^+ load, whereas the tubular secretion of H^+ in exchange for Na^+ is thought to occur via the rapid (within 1–2 min) stimulation of a Na^+-H^+ antiporter in these cells. Recent evidence indicates that this latter

effect may be non-genomically mediated following the interaction of aldosterone with specific surface membrane receptors (insensitive to *spironolactone* or *canrenoate*). The involvement of intracellular *inositol 1,4,5-trisphosphate (IP₃)* in mediating these effects has also been suggested.

The principal steps involved in the action of mineralocorticoids are summarized in Figure 3.6.

☞ The presence of the local enzyme *11-β-hydroxysteroid dehydrogenase (11-HSD)* in aldosterone-sensitive tissues ensures mineralocorticoid specificity of the intracellular type I mineralocorticoid receptor, by catalysing the conversion of circulating cortisol and corticosterone to their receptor-inactive analogues cortisone and 11-dehydrocorticosterone respectively (aldosterone itself is a poor substrate for 11-HSD). This effectively prevents glucocorticoids from reaching mineralocorticoid receptors and thus confers aldosterone specificity. In patients that lack 11-HSD, or where the activity of the enzyme has been compromised (due to excess ingestion of liquorice!), 'protection' of the mineralocorticoid receptors is lost, allowing cortisol to exert mineralocorticoid effects in the kidney. Such individuals show symptoms of mineralocorticoid excess (see below) such as *Na^+ retention, hypertension* and a *low plasma K^+ level (hypokalaemia)* that may be treated by administration of *spironolactone*.

Control of Release of Aldosterone

Although ACTH does transiently stimulate some aldosterone release, and is important in the tonic maintenance of the *zona glomerulosa*, it is *not* considered a major factor in the long-term control of aldosterone production and secretion. The release is, instead mainly influenced by the renin-angiotensin system and the plasma sodium and potassium concentrations.

Renin-Angiotensin System. Renin is a proteolytic enzyme released by specialized *juxtaglomerular cells* (situated within the afferent arteriolar walls of the kidney) when there is a *fall* in renal blood pressure and an excessive reduction in circulating blood volume (e.g. during haemorrhage, salt or water loss). Circulating renin promotes the production of an inactive decapeptide **angiotensin I** from an $α_2$-globulin precursor **angiotensinogen** (derived from the liver). Angiotensin I is rapidly converted in the lung and plasma (via the *angiotensin-converting enzyme; ACE*) to the active octapeptide **angiotensin II**, which directly stimulates the synthesis and release of aldosterone from the *zona glomerulosa* of the adrenal cortex. Angiotensin II also has a potent, direct vasoconstrictor action that helps to maintain the blood pressure of the arterial circulation under extreme conditions, and a further important central effect (via the

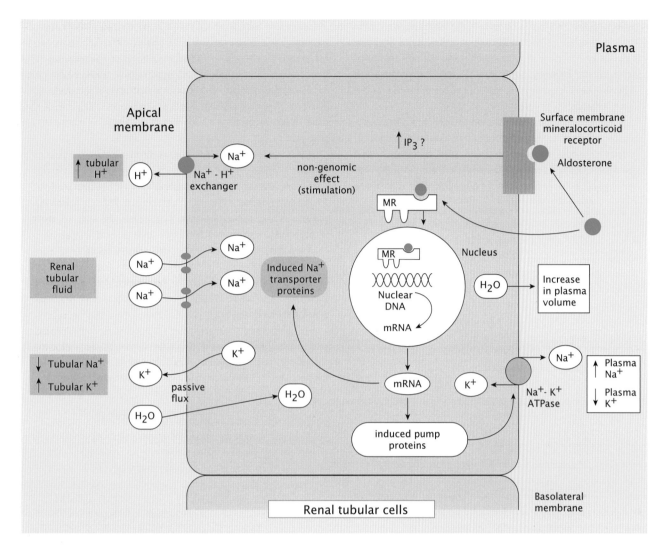

Figure 3.6. Mechanism of action of aldosterone on renal tubular Na^+ reabsorption and K^+/H^+ excretion. Binding of aldosterone to an intracellular *mineralocorticoid receptor protein (MR)*, followed by translocation of the complex to the nucleus and binding with nuclear DNA, induces the *de novo* synthesis of Na^+ channel proteins that facilitate the transfer of Na^+ across the luminal membrane and also Na^+/K^+-ATPase molecules that pump Na^+ into the interstitial fluid. K^+ efflux may occur passively in exchange for Na^+, whereas secretion of H^+ (via the Na^+-H^+ antiporter) may be stimulated by a *rapid* non-genomic mechanism involving a surface membrane mineralocorticoid receptor (linked to intracellular IP_3 [inositol 1,4,5-trisphosphate] generation).

subfornical organ) to control water intake (*dipsogenic effect*); [ACE inhibitor compounds such as **captopril** (*Capoten*) and **enalapril maleate** (*Innovace*) are currently being used in the treatment of hypertension and heart failure].

Circulating angiotensin II is degraded by angiotensinase enzymes (e.g. *glutamyl aminopeptidise A*) to **angiotensin III** (heptapeptide) [and ultimately to **angiotensin IV** (hexapeptide)], which has less potent, though similar vasoconstrictor and aldosterone-releasing actions to angiotensin II.

☞ Two main types of specific cell surface angiotensin II receptor have been described, termed AT_1 and AT_2, with two subtypes of AT_1 (AT_{1A} and AT_{1B}); the angiotensin II receptors of the adrenal cortex are mainly of the AT_{1B} subtype, linked through activation of *phospholipase C* to the intracellular generation of IP_3, release of Ca^{2+} from internal stores, and consequent stimulation of aldosterone synthesis (involving inner mitochondrial transport of cholesterol). AT_{1A} receptors are the predominant type found in the kidney, blood vessel walls and the brain; AT_2 receptors are also present in the brain and other peripheral tissues, but their functional role has not been clearly defined. Highly selective AT_1 receptor antagonists **losartan potassium** (*Cozaar*) and **Valsartan** (*Diovan*) have recently been introduced for the treatment of hypertension.

Angiotensin IV has been shown to bind to a pharmacologically distinct type of angiotensin receptor (termed AT_4), particularly concentrated on aortic and coronary vessel endothelial cells, as well as mammalian heart, adrenal gland and brain; the physiological role of angiotensin IV in these tissues however, is unknown.

Plasma Na+ and K+ Concentrations. Either a large *decrease* (>20 mEq/l) in plasma Na+ or a small *increase* (ca. 1 mEq/l) in plasma K+ concentration stimulates the synthesis and release of aldosterone by a direct action on the biosynthetic enzymes in the adrenal cortex.

Clinical Disorders

Mineralocorticoid Hyposecretion

Isolated deficiency in aldosterone production (*hypoaldosteronism*) due to adrenal enzyme defects is very rare, but it may occur for example, as a consequence of renal disease due to *diabetes mellitus* (see Chapter 5) or in patients with AIDS. The general symptoms of mineralocorticoid deficiency i.e. increased Na+/H_2O excretion, hyperkalaemia (high plasma K+), hypotension and metabolic acidosis would also be seen in conjunction with those of glucocorticoid lack in cases of adrenal insufficiency (e.g. Addison's disease), treated by replacement therapy.

Mineralocorticoid Hypersecretion

Aldosterone excess (*hyperaldosteronism*) may be divided into two types:

Primary Aldosteronism (Conn's Syndrome). This is usually caused by a bilateral adrenal hyperplasia (abnormal enlargement) or small tumour (adenoma) of the adrenal *zona glomerulosa*. Patients exhibit *hypertension* (due to Na+ and H_2O retention, without peripheral oedema) and a *low plasma K+ level (hypokalaemia)*; *muscle weakness*, fatigue and cardiac dysrhythmias; a mild *metabolic alkalosis* may also be present;

Plasma renin levels are characteristically *low* in this condition.

Diagnosis is made by demonstration of a *high plasma or urine aldosterone level*, in conjunction with a *low level of plasma renin*; blood volume expansion by saline loading, would fail to suppress the high aldosterone level.

Treatment would involve the surgical removal of the tumour responsible for the disorder, or long-term administration of an aldosterone receptor antagonist e.g. **spironolactone**. The latter would also be used in the control of patients prior to surgery.

Secondary Aldosteronism. This is caused by an abnormally increased *renin* release, and therefore raised levels of *angiotensin II*. Patients may have peripheral oedema.

Some possible causes include:

- Poor renal perfusion e.g. in renal artery stenosis;
- Malignant hypertension (i.e. hypertension associated with progressive renal failure due to renal arteriolar necrosis);
- Renal tumour of the juxtaglomerular cells;
- Excessive Na+ and H_2O loss during diuretic therapy (most common cause) or dietary Na+ deprivation;
- Congestive heart failure or liver cirrhosis.

Treatment of the underlying cause of the abnormal renin-angiotensin system activation should be attempted, coupled with administration of **spironolactone** for long-term management. ∎

Review Questions

Question 1: State the location of the adrenal glands and explain briefly, the morphology of the medulla and outer cortex regions.

Question 2: List the major secretions of each cortical area.

Question 3: Define the terms glucocorticoid and mineralocorticoid and name the naturally secreted hormones of each group.

Question 4: Name the plasma precursor from which all steroids are derived.

Question 5: Under what conditions may the secretion of sex steroids from the adrenal cortex become physiologically significant?

Question 6: Describe the mechanisms controlling cortisol release; what do understand by the circadian rhythm of ACTH/cortisol secretion?

Question 7: Describe the main effects of cortisol on:
(a) carbohydrate metabolism
(b) protein metabolism
(c) fat (lipid) metabolism.

Question 8: Describe how cortisol protects the body from unfavourable stresses.

Question 9: Explain how glucocorticoids at therapeutic doses, produce antiinflammatory and immunosuppressive effects.

Question 10: Give examples of some commonly used synthetic glucocorticoids.

Question 11: Outline how glucocorticoids and mineralocorticoids exert their effects via intracellular receptors.

Question 12: Describe the causes, symptoms and treatment of Addison's disease.

Question 13: Explain why prolonged corticosteroid therapy can also lead to hyposecretion of cortisol.

Question 14: Describe the causes, symptoms and treatment of Cushing's syndrome.

Question 15: What is the overnight dexamethasone suppression test? How may this test be useful in the diagnosis of Cushing's syndrome? Would this test be able to distinguish between pituitary-dependent Cushing's disease and hypercortisolism due to ectopic ACTH secretion?

Question 16: Describe the main effects of aldosterone on Na^+/H_2O excretion.

Question 17: Give examples of a clinically useful mineralocorticoid and an aldosterone antagonist.

Question 18: Describe the mechanisms controlling aldosterone release, mentioning:
(a) the renin angiotensin system
(b) the effects of plasma Na^+/K^+ concentration.

Question 19: What are ACE inhibitors? Give examples of some currently available compounds, and their therapeutic uses.

Question 20: Describe the causes, symptoms and treatment of Conn's syndrome.

Clinical Case Studies

Patient 1

A 28 year old female was referred to a hospital Endocrinology Department with amenorrhoea of six months duration, weight gain, an increase in facial hair growth and muscle weakness, with occasional calf cramps. Clinical examination revealed a weight of 17 stone (238 lb; 108 kg) with a blood pressure of 160/90 mmHg. She had a rounded face with marked hirsutism (prominent soft hair growth on the upper lip and chin area); she also had several bruise patches (ecchymoses) over her extremities, particularly her legs. The abdomen was protuberant and supraclavicular and dorsal fat pads were enlarged. Examination of her heart and chest was normal. Neurological examination was also normal. She had no visual symptoms.

Laboratory tests revealed that her full blood count (FBC), urinalysis and electrolytes were normal; blood chemistry however, showed a blood glucose of 8.3 mmol/l (150 mg/dl). An oral glucose tolerance test (see Chapter 5) indicated a mild diabetes. In the *overnight dexamethasone suppression test*, plasma cortisol measured at 8 a.m., following oral administration of *1 mg dexamethasone* at 12 p.m. the previous night, was 23 µg/dl (normal <5 µg/dl). Urinary free cortisol was 230 µg/24 hours (normal 20–100 µg/24 h), and the plasma ACTH level at 8 a.m. was 150 pg/ml (normal 40–100 pg/ml). The patient then underwent a standard *low dose (2 mg/day for 2 days) oral dexamethasone suppression test* which failed to alter the plasma cortisol level; a *high dose (8 mg/day for 2 days) dexamethasone test* however, resulted in a >60% reduction in plasma cortisol from the basal pre-test level, indicating a high set-point but intact negative feedback inhibitory mechanism.

An adrenal CT scan appeared normal, but an MRI (magnetic resonance image) of the head revealed an 8 mm pituitary microadenoma.

Question 1: What is the most likely diagnosis in this patient?

Question 2: What is the basis of the laboratory screening tests ordered for the patient, and what results would you expect if the diagnosis is correct?

Question 3: What treatment would you recommend for this condition?

Answer 1: The patient's symptoms of rounded 'moon' face, increased facial hair and lack of menstruation (virilization by adrenal androgens), trunk obesity, 'buffalo hump', bruises, mild hypertension and impaired glucose tolerance are characteristic of *chronic excess glucocorticoid secretion (Cushing's syndrome)*.

The latter may arise as a consequence of an ACTH-secreting pituitary adenoma, an adrenal cortical adenoma, or ectopic secretion of ACTH or CRH. Long-term treatment with exogenous glucocorticoids may also lead to Cushing's syndrome, and remains the most common cause of this condition in clinical practice.

Answer 2: Measurement of 24 hour urinary free cortisol, or an *overnight dexamethasone suppression test* remain the two most often used initial screening tests for Cushing's syndrome. Twenty-four hour urinary samples are useful in providing an 'average' of a day's hormone secretion; random cortisol measurements are of little value. In the alternative *low dose dexamethasone suppression test*, administration of dexamethasone (0.5 mg q.d.s. for 2 days) will suppress adrenal cortisol production in normal individuals but not in subjects with Cushing's syndrome. Following a *high dose dexamethasone suppression test* (2 mg q.d.s. for 2 days), cortisol secretion would be suppressed if the Cushing's syndrome is pituitary-dependent (termed Cushing's *disease*), [as in the above case], but not if it arises from excess ectopic ACTH or CRH, or an adrenal tumour. For this patient, a CT scan confirmed the presence of a pituitary (ACTH-secreting) adenoma. Note that the plasma level of ACTH was correspondingly high; a low (or undetectable) ACTH level (<0.01 pg/ml) would have been indicative of non-ACTH dependent disease.

Answer 3: Transsphenoidal surgery is the treatment of choice for pituitary-dependent Cushing's disease. When surgery is inappropriate, the aromatase enzyme inhibitor *aminoglutethimide (250 mg–1 g daily)*, may be used to block adrenal steroid synthesis. In children, external irradiation therapy is equally effective as surgery or even superior.

The patient underwent transsphenoidal adenomectomy with total amelioration of her Cushingoid symptoms, and normalization of blood pressure, menstrual periods and blood glucose within four months following surgery. She remained asymptomatic with normal plasma cortisol and blood glucose thereafter.

Patient 2

A 39 year old female presented at the hospital outpatient's clinic with a history of dizziness (particularly on standing), increasing fatigue and muscle cramps and some loss of scalp and body hair (underarm, pubic). The symptoms had worsened in the last 4 months, during which she had lost about 1 stone (14 lb; 6.4 kg) in weight. She had no prior medical history. Clinical examination revealed a supine (lying down) blood pressure of 110/65 mmHg, with a marked postural hypotension (30 mmHg on standing); there was distinctive freckling of the face and increased pigmentation skin creases around the palms, elbows and knees, and over the buccal mucosa in the mouth. There were also three small areas of vitiligo over her back.

Laboratory investigation revealed a normal full blood count (FBC) and urinalysis. Blood chemistry however, gave a serum Na^+ of 129 mmol/l (normal 135–145 mmol/l), K^+ 5.8 mmol/l (normal 3.5–5.0 mmol/l) and blood glucose of 3.2 mM (normal 3.6–6.4 mmol/l). Chest X-ray and thyroid function tests were normal. Deep tendon reflexes were also normal. The plasma cortisol level measured at 8 a.m. was 2.1 µg/dl (normal 5–20 µg/dl) with a concomitant ACTH level of 1200 pg/ml (normal 40–100 pg/ml). Plasma aldosterone at 8 a.m. was 1.8 ng/dl (normal 6–30 ng/dl, upright). After a *short ACTH stimulation test*, the plasma cortisol level remained unchanged one hour post-test.

Question 1:   *What is the most likely cause of the patients's symptoms?*
Question 2:   *What are the diagnostic criteria for the condition?*
Question 3:   *How is the disorder treated?*

Answer   1:   This is a classical presentation of *primary hypoadrenalism (Addison's disease)*, confirmed by the low plasma cortisol and aldosterone levels along with a high level of ACTH. The condition is most commonly caused by autoimmune damage to both adrenal glands; however, adrenal damage arising from infections, sarcoidal or tubercular infiltrations or acute haemorrhage may also lead to adrenal insufficiency. Use of drugs interfering with steroid synthesis (*aminoglutethimide*) or action will also result in a clinical picture of hypoadrenalism. The symptoms of dizziness, fatigue, weight loss and muscle cramps result from a combined lack of cortisol and aldosterone action on brain and muscle cells. Aldosterone deficiency causes loss of total body Na^+/H_2O, a reduction in blood volume and postural hypotension; this is accompanied by a decreased K^+ excretion, leading to hyperkalaemia. Scalp alopecia (hair loss) and vitiligo (skin depigmentation) most likely result from an associated autoimmune attack of hair follicles and skin melanocytes respectively; loss of axillary and pubic hair is due to lack of adrenal androgens, normally important for growth of body hair in females. The increased skin pigmentation and face freckling are caused by the melanocyte stimulating (MSH-like) action of excess ACTH.

Answer   2:   Diagnosis of Addison's disease is made by documentation of low plasma cortisol and aldosterone levels with concurrent high ACTH levels; the titre of *anti-adrenal antibodies* in the serum would also be expected to be high. The lack of adrenal response to ACTH was confirmed by the *short ACTH stimulation test* in which 250 µg of synthetic ACTH (*tetracosactrin*) is administered intravenously over 2 min, and plasma cortisol levels measured at 30 and 60 mins following the injection. Normally a peak level of 18 µg/dl or more is seen during the test. Patients with adrenal failure are unable to achieve this level.

Answer 3: Treatment of Addison's disease involves combined replacement doses of a glucocorticoid and a mineralocorticoid taken for life. On diagnosis of primary hypoadrenalism, the patient was started on *hydrocortisone (25 µg/ day)* and *fludrocortisone (0.1 mg/day)* replacement therapy. The patient became totally asymptomatic within ten days, but was advised to double her glucocorticoid dose during any period of stress (in an attempt to mimic the normal physiological response).

Patient 3

A 52 year old man was admitted to the hospital Endocrinology Division for evaluation of hypertension of four years duration, with progressive muscular weakness and muscle cramps. The patient had been treated with various antihypertensive medications without significant improvement. His history was negative for any other medical illness, and there was no family background of hypertension or neuromuscular disease. He had been placed on potassium supplements about two years ago, but he did not know why. Lately, he had stopped taking potassium. He was not taking any other medications. Clinical examination revealed hypertension (195/105 mmHg; supine) and an early systolic ejection murmur in the aortic area. There was no peripheral oedema.

Laboratory investigation revealed a normal FBC and urinalysis; blood chemistry gave a serum Na^+ of 149 mmol/l (normal 135–145 mmol/l) and a serum K^+ of 2.6 mmol/l (normal 3.5–5.0 mmol/l). Further investigation showed normal 24 hour levels of urinary free catecholamines, metadrenaline and vanillylmandelic acid (VMA). His 8 a.m. plasma cortisol and 24 hour urinary free cortisol levels were normal; however, he showed a plasma aldosterone of 35 ng/dl (normal 6–30 ng/dl, upright) with a concurrent plasma renin activity of 0.6 ng/ml/hour (normal 1.3–4.0 ng/ml/hour). The renin activity did not increase after slow intravenous administration of *frusemide* (40 mg) and 4 hours of ambulation (upright posture). A CT scan of the abdomen showed a round and solitary tumour (2.5 cm diameter) in the left adrenal gland.

Question 1: *What are the common causes of endocrine hypertension?*
Question 2: *What is the most likely diagnosis in this patient, and how may the condition be treated?*

Answer 1: The main causes of endocrine hypertension include an adrenal medullary tumour (*phaeochromocytoma*), Cushing's syndrome, mineralocorticoid excess (primary aldosteronism, congenital adrenal hyperplasia), hyperthyroidism, acromegaly and hypercalcaemia. Urinary excretion of the adrenaline/noradrenaline metabolites, metadrenaline/normetadrenaline and VMA would be markedly increased in patients with phaeochromocytoma.

Answer 2: A combination of chronic Na^+ retention (resulting in hypertension) and an unprovoked hypokalaemia (typically resistant to potassium supplementa- tion — causing muscle weakness and cramps) suggests a possible *hyperaldosteronism*. A characteristic of *primary hyperaldosteronism (Conn's syndrome)* is the combination of a high plasm aldosterone level with suppressed plasma renin activity. An increase in renin secretion by the kidney juxtaglomerular cells would normally be expected following a stimulus that reduces renal perfusion pressure, decreases plasma volume or causes Na$^+$ depletion (e.g. a diuretic). In the present case, the ongoing hypertension and Na$^+$ retention caused by excess (non-suppressible) aldosterone secretion continues to depress normal renin activity, despite a diuretic challenge by the 'loop' diuretic *frusemide*.

Treatment depends upon the type of underlying pathology. In this patient, the diagnosis of an aldosterone producing adenoma (*aldosteronoma*) was confirmed, and he underwent a left adrenalectomy with resolution of his hypokalaemia and hypertension [the aldosterone antagonist *spironolactone* may also be used to manage patients prior to surgery]. He remains asymptomatic at three years post-surgery.

UK/USA Drugs — Trade names		
	UK	**USA**
ACTH/ ACTH analogue		
ACTH		Acthar/Cortrosyn
Tetracosactrin	Syncathen	
Glucocorticoids		
Beclomethasone	Propaderm	Beclovent/Beconase
Betamethasone	Betnelan	Celestone
	Betnovate	Lotrisone
Dexamethasone	Decadron	Decadron/Hexadrol
Fluocinolone	Synalar	Synalar/Fluonid
Hydrocortisone	Hydrocortistab	Cortef/Hydrocortone
Prednisolone	Prednesol	Delta-cortef
	Deltastab	Blephamide
	Precortisyl	Prelone
Triamcinolone	Adcortyl	Aristocort
Glucocorticoid-mineralocorticoid		
Cortisone	Cortisyl	Cortone
Mineralocorticoid		
Fludrocortisone	Florinef	Florinef
Aldosterone antagonist		
Spironolactone	Aldactone	Aldactone
Steroid synthesis inhibitor		
Aminoglutethimide	Orimeten	Cytadren

References

Books

- **Aron DC, Tyrrell JB.** (1994). Glucocorticoids & adrenal androgens. In *Basic & Clinical Endocrinology*, edited by FS Greenspan, JD Baxter, 4th ed. Appleton & Lange, Connecticut, pp. 307–346
- **Chandrasoma P, Taylor CR.** (1991). The adrenal cortex & medulla. In *Concise Pathology*, 1st ed. Prentice-Hall, USA, pp. 864–876
- **Fitzgerald PA, Copeland PM.** (1992). Adrenal disorders. In *Handbook of Clinical Endocrinology*, edited by PA Fitzgerald, 2nd ed. Prentice-Hall, USA, pp. 227–287
- **Fletcher RF.** (1987). Adrenal. In *Lecture Notes on Endocrinology*, 4th ed, Blackwell Scientific Publications, Oxford, pp. 144–168
- **Ganong WF.** (1995). The adrenal medulla & adrenal cortex. In *Review of Medical Physiology*, 17th ed, Appleton & Lange, Connecticut, pp. 327–351
- **Genuth SM.** (1993). The adrenal glands. In *Physiology*, edited by RM Berne, MN Levy, 3rd ed. Mosby-Year Book, Inc, USA, pp. 949–979
- **Goodman HM.** (1988). Adrenal glands. In *Basic Medical Endocrinology*, Raven Press, New York, pp. 71–113
- **Guyton AC, Hall JE.** (1996). The adrenocortical hormones. In *Textbook of Medical Physiology*, 9th ed. WB Saunders Company, USA, pp. 957–970
- **Hedge GA, Colby HD, Goodman RL.** (1987). Adrenal cortex. In *Clinical Endocrine Physiology*, WB. Saunders Co, Philadelphia, pp. 127–159
- **Junqueira LC, Carneiro J, Long JA.** (1986). Adrenals & other endocrine glands. In *Basic Histology*, 5th ed, Lange Medical Publications, Connecticut, pp. 446–467
- **Kaplan NM.** (1988). The adrenal glands. In *Textbook of Endocrine Physiology*, edited by JE. Griffin, SR Ojeda. Oxford University Press, New York, pp. 245–272
- **Laurence DR, Bennett PN.** (1992). Endocrinology I: adrenal corticosteroids, antagonists, corticotrophin. In *Clinical Pharmacology*, Churchill Livingstone, pp. 549–563
- **Magiakou M-A, Chrousos GP.** (1994). Diagnosis and treatment of Cushing's disease. In *The Pituitary Gland*, edited by H Imura, 2nd ed. Raven Press Ltd, New York, pp. 491–508
- **Playfair JHL.** (1990). Cell-mediated immune responses. In *Immunology at a glance*, 4th ed, Blackwell Scientific Publications, Oxford, Chapters 6 and 19
- **Rang HP, Dale MM, Ritter JM.** (1995). *Pharmacology*, 3rd ed, Churchill Livingstone, Chapters 11 and 21
- **Schimmer BP, Parker KL.** (1996). Adrenocorticotrophic hormone; adrenocortical steroids and their synthetic analogs. In *Goodman & Gilman's The Pharmacological Basis of Therapeutics*, edited by JG Hardman, LE Limbird. A Goodman, Gilman et al, 9th ed. McGraw-Hill, USA, pp. 1459–1485
- **Whitby LG, Percy-Robb IW, Smith AF.** (1984). Steroid hormones. In *Lecture Notes on Clinical Chemistry*, 3rd ed, Blackwell Scientific Publications, Oxford, pp. 354–386

Journal Articles

- **Barnes PJ, Adcock I.** (1993). Anti-inflammatory actions of steroids: molecular mechanisms. *Trends in Pharmacol Sci*, 14, 436–441
- **Capponi AM, Python CP, Rossier MF.** (1994). Molecular basis of angiotensin II action on mineralocorticoid synthesis. *Endocrine*, 2, 579–586
- **Cato ACB, Wade E.** (1996). Molecular mechanisms of anti-inflammatory action of glucocorticoids. *BioEssays*, 18, 371–378
- **Edwards CRW,** *et al.* (1988). 11β-hydroxysteroid dehydrogenase-tissue specific protector of the mineralocorticoid receptor. *Lancet* ii, 986–989
- **Funder JW.** (1993). Aldosterone action. *Annu Rev Physiol*, 55, 115–130
- **Funder JW,** *et al.* (1988). Mineralocorticoid action: target tissue specificity is enzyme, not receptor, mediated. *Science*, 242, 583–585
- **Kakouris H, Eddie LW, Summers RJ.** (1993). Aldosterone-specific membrane receptors and related rapid, non-genomic effects. *Trends in Pharmacol Sci*, 14, 1–6
- **Müller J.** (1995). Aldosterone: The minority hormone of the adrenal cortex. *Steroids*, 60, 2–9
- **Munck, A, Naray Fejes Toth A.** (1994). Glucocorticoids and stress: Permissive and suppressive actions. *Ann NY Acad Sci*, 746, 115–130
- **O'Banion MK, Winn VD, Young DA.** (1992). cDNA cloning and functional activity of a glucocorticoid-regulated inflammatory cyclooxygenase. *Proc Natl Acad Sci USA*, 89, 4888–4892
- **Orti E, Bodwell JE, Munck A.** (1992). Phosphorylation of steroid hormone receptors. *Endocrine Rev*, 13, 105–128
- **Power RF, Conneely OM, O'Malley BW.** (1992). New insights into activation of the steroid hormone receptor superfamily. *Trends in Pharmacol Sci*, 13, 318–323
- **Pratt WB.** (1993). The role of heat shock proteins in regulating the function, folding and trafficking of the glucocorticoid receptor. *J Biol Chem*, 268, 21455–21458
- **Schleimer RP.** (1993). An overview of glucocorticoid anti-inflammatory actions. *Eur J Clin Pharmacol*, 45, S3–S7
- **Smith DF, Toft DO.** (1993). Steroid receptors and their associated proteins. *Molec Endocrinol*, 7, 4–11
- **Stewart PM, Wallace AM,** *et al.* (1987). Mineralocorticoid activity of liquorice: 11β-hydroxysteroid dehydrogenase deficiency comes of age. *Lancet*, 2, 821–824
- **Wehling M.** (1994). Nongenomic actions of steroid hormones. *Trends Endocrinol Metab*, 5, 347–353
- **Wehling M.** (1997). Specific, nongenomic actions of steroid hormones. *Annu Rev Physiol*, 59, 365–393
- **Wehling M, Eisen C, Christ M.** (1993). Membrane receptors for aldosterone: a new concept of nongenomic mineralocorticoid action. *News in Physiol Sci*, 8, 241–244
- **Weinberger C, Bradley DJ.** (1990). Gene regulation by receptors binding lipid-soluble substances. *Annu Rev Physiol*, 52, 823–840

4 The Thyroid Gland

Structure and Histology

The thyroid gland develops embryologically as an epithelial invagination from the base of the foetal tongue. It consists of two large lobes (normally weighing ca. 15–20 g) lying on both sides of the trachea, just beneath the larynx (voice box), connected by a narrow strand of thyroid tissue called the *isthmus* (Figure 4.1A); a small pyramidal extension of tissue upwards from the isthmus is also sometimes present. The gland receives a profuse blood supply through the thyroid arteries, and is also richly innervated by fibres of the autonomic nervous system, although the role played by these nerves in the control of thyroid blood flow and function seems minimal. The whole gland is enveloped by a capsule of fibrous connective tissue.

Histology

Thyroid tissue is composed of numerous closed spherical *follicles* (ca. 200–300 µm in diameter), each comprising of a rim of simple cuboidal epithelial cells surrounding a mass of colloidal storage protein called *thyroglobulin* (a 670 kDa glycoprotein). The height of the cuboidal epithelium can vary according to the functional state of the gland: thus, when the gland is relatively inactive, the colloidal mass is large and the surrounding follicular cells are flattened, whereas under hyperactive conditions, the follicular lumen decreases in size, and the endocrine cells become columnar in appearance. Fingers of loose connective tissue, containing blood vessels, lymphatics and nerve fibres, separate the follicles into several functional lobules. Lying in between the thyroid follicles are groups of separate larger epithelial cells, the *parafollicular C cells*, responsible for the secretion of a peptide hormone **calcitonin**, involved in the control of calcium metabolism (see Chapter 7). C-cells may also be present in the follicular epithelium, but never border the follicular lumen (Figure 4.1B).

Biosynthesis and Release of Thyroid Hormones

The two active hormones secreted by the thyroid, are iodinated derivatives of the amino acid *tyrosine*; these are **thyroxine (T_4;** about 90% of output) containing four iodine

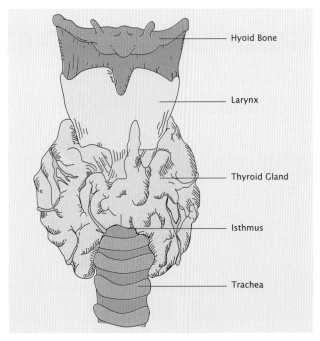

Figure 4.1(A). Anterior view of the human thyroid gland.

- Hyoid Bone
- Larynx
- Thyroid Gland
- Isthmus
- Trachea

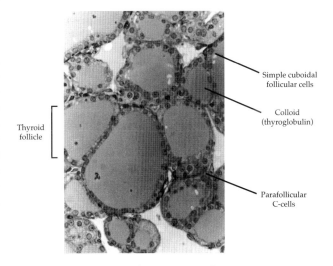

Thyroid follicle

Simple cuboidal follicular cells

Colloid (thyroglobulin)

Parafollicular C-cells

Figure 4.1(B). Histological appearance of a transverse section of the thyroid gland. Each thyroid follicle (lined with simple cuboidal epithelial cells) is filled with thyroglobulin storage protein (colloid); note the variable size of the follicles. Calcitonin-producing parafollicular cells are present in between the follicles (magnification × 40).

atoms, and **triiodothyronine** (T_3; about 10% of output) containing three iodine atoms. The term 'thyroid hormone' thus encompasses both T_3 and T_4.

Inorganic iodine is concentrated within the thyroid follicular cells by a highly efficient, active iodide pump mechanism that removes it from the thyroid blood supply. A wide range of anions can compete with iodide for the carrier system, and can thereby inhibit the activity of the iodide pump e.g. *perchlorate (ClO_4^-), thiocyanate (SCN^-)* or *pertechnetate (TcO_4^-)* (Tc = Technetium).

☞ Radioactive pertechnetate administered in the form of an isotonic injection solution (sodium pertechnetate [^{99m}Tc] injection BP) is widely used clinically as a radioactive label in thyroid (and also brain) diagnostic scanning procedures. Tc-99m is a metastable radionuclide formed by the radioactive decay of molybdenum-99.

The processes involved in thyroid hormone synthesis and release may be summarized as follows:

1. Accumulated iodide is rapidly oxidized to free iodine by a *thyroid peroxidase* enzyme at the apical surface of the follicular cell, and is then immediately incorporated into the 3- and 5-ring positions of the tyrosine molecules to form **monoiodotyrosine (MIT)** and **diiodotyrosine (DIT)** respectively.

2. Coupling of MIT and DIT via an ether linkage then occurs (involving the same thyroid peroxidase enzyme) to form the active hormones **T_3 (3,5,3'-triiodothyronine)** and **T_4 (3,5,3',5'-tetraiodothyronine or thyroxine)**. Small amounts (<1%) of the 3,3',5'-triiodothyronine derivative (reverse T_3 or rT_3) are also synthesized, but this has no significant biological activity (Figure 4.2). Under conditions of starvation or severe illness, larger amounts of rT_3 may be produced relative to T_3.

3. During iodination and coupling, the tyrosyl residues remain covalently linked to thyroglobulin molecules at the apical border; (the large thyroglobulin precursor polypeptide is produced continuously as secretory vesicles by the follicular cells, and exocytosed into the colloid through the apical membrane). The thyroid hormones remain in this stored form within the colloid, until they are secreted.

4. Under the influence of the thyroid stimulating hormone **thyrotrophin (TSH)**, resorption and proteolysis of the stored thyroglobulin-hormone complex within the follicular cells leads to the release of active hormones (ca. 20:1, T_4:T_3) by diffusion from the basal surface into the local capillary blood supply. Thyroxine is then deiodinated in peripheral tissues (e.g. liver and kidney) to yield the more active T_3 (ca. 10 times more potent); MIT, DIT and released iodide are re-utilized for hormone synthesis by the gland (Figure 4.3). Only minimal amounts

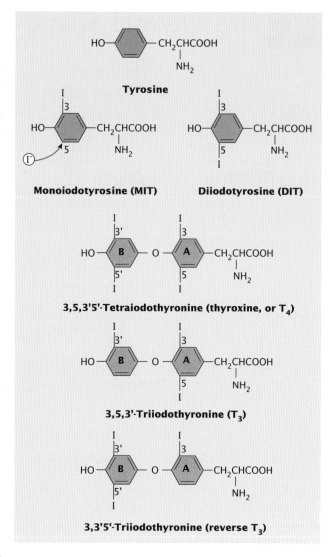

Figure 4.2. Chemical structure of the thyroid hormones and their intermediate precursors. Numbers indicate positions of iodine atoms in the molecule.

of the free thyroglobulin normally escape from the follicles to reach the blood stream.

☞ The presence of iodine atoms in the thyroid hormone molecule does not appear to be essential for biological activity, since these can be replaced by other bulky/hydrophobic groupings to yield equally (or more) active analogues.

In the bloodstream, T_3 and T_4 are extensively bound (>99%) to plasma proteins (principally *thyroxine binding globulin [TBG], thyroxine binding prealbumin* and *albumin*); it should however be noted, that only the free unbound hormones are biologically active on their target cells. T_3 is less avidly bound by plasma proteins than T_4.

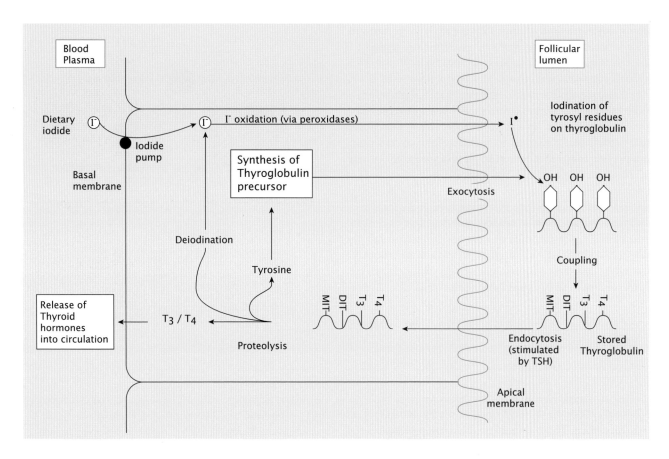

Figure 4.3. Synthesis and release of thyroid hormones (T$_3$ and T$_4$) by the thyroid follicular cell. Dietary iodide, pumped actively through the basal membrane, is oxidized and attached to thyroglobulin tyrosyl residues at the apical surface. Internal coupling of iodotyrosines leads to T$_3$/T$_4$ production. Endocytosis and proteolysis of thyroglobulin releases thyroid hormones into the circulating blood. MIT, DIT and tyrosine are re-utilized for synthesis.

Control of Release

Synthesis and release of thyroid hormone is controlled by pituitary **thyrotrophin (TSH)**, which interacts with specific receptors on the basal membrane of the follicular cells to cause an increase in intracellular cAMP and subsequent activation of protein kinase A (see Figure 1.2). TSH also stimulates the active iodide pump process by inducing the synthesis and insertion of new carrier molecules in the basal membrane. Release of TSH is, in turn, stimulated by hypothalamic TRH and regulated by negative feedback effects exerted by free circulating thyroid hormones (principally T$_3$) on the anterior pituitary gland (see Figure 2.4).

Thyroid Hormones

Thyroid hormones increase the *basal metabolic rate (BMR)* (a measure of O$_2$ consumption) in virtually all tissues of the body. They stimulate the synthesis of specific proteins involved in *calorigenesis* (heat production) and also influence protein, carbohydrate and fat metabolism.

Calorigenesis

Thyroid hormones increase O$_2$ consumption in all tissues except the brain, testes, anterior pituitary and spleen, which results in increased heat production (through the splitting of ATP molecules) and is therefore important in the process of thermoregulation in a cold environment. It is now believed that this effect (which has a typically long latent period of 4–5 days) may be mediated partly through the synthesis of new Na$^+$, K$^+$-ATPase (sodium pump) molecules in the cell membranes, and partly via a direct (non-genomic) activation of oxidative phosphorylation in liver mitochondria.

Influence on Metabolism

Carbohydrate metabolism is stimulated both directly (via an increase in gastrointestinal glucose absorption and the synthesis of specific metabolic enzymes) and indirectly by an increase in tissue sensitivity to catecholamines, insulin and growth hormone. The net result is an increase in gluconeogenesis and glycogenolysis in the liver, and glucose utilization by fat, liver and muscle cells. Enhanced glycogenolysis is particularly evident in patients with hyperthyroidism (see below).

Protein metabolism (both resynthesis and degradation) is stimulated when thyroid hormone levels are low; however, at abnormally high levels, protein breakdown predominates (particularly marked in muscle), leading to significant weight loss and elevation in plasma amino acid levels.

Fat metabolism is generally stimulated, but lipolysis is favoured, along with an increased oxidation of free fatty acids. Part of this lipolytic effect is due to potentiation of catecholamine activity on adipose tissue (a β-adrenoceptor effect). Plasma cholesterol is lowered by thyroid hormones, through an indirect facilitation of liver cholesterol uptake from the blood (increased synthesis of *low-density lipoprotein (LDL) receptors* in the liver cell membranes).

Maturation of the Central Nervous System (CNS)

Thyroid hormones are essential for normal CNS development during late foetal and early postnatal life; the optimal growth of cortical and cerebellar neurones, and the adequate myelination of nerve fibres is vitally dependent on their presence. Their absence or deficiency *in utero* or at birth, if not diagnosed early and promptly treated with thyroid hormone replacement, invariably causes irreversible mental retardation (*cretinism*).

Skeletal Growth and Maturation

The actions of thyroid hormone are generally synergistic with those of *growth hormone (GH)*; thyroid hormone is thus essential for normal bone growth and maturation, and the eventual development of normal adult stature. Normal amounts of thyroid hormone are also necessary for proper functioning of the nervous and cardiovascular systems, the gastrointestinal tract, as well as for regular development of the teeth, skin and hair follicles.

Mechanism of Action of Thyroid Hormones

Being lipophilic molecules, free (unbound) T_3 or T_4 are able to enter target cells freely by passive diffusion; in addition, active transport of T_3 and T_4 into some cells can also occur via specific carrier proteins. Upon cell entry, T_4 is immediately monodeiodinated to form the more active T_3, or the inactive rT_3 derivatives; (T_4 is therefore regarded as a *prohormone* in this respect). Like the steroid hormones, the effects of T_3 are mediated by an interaction with specific high affinity *thyroid hormone receptors (TRs)* located in the

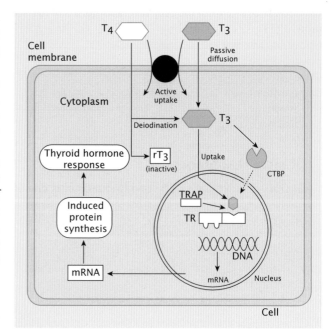

Figure 4.4. Proposed intracellular mechanism of action of the thyroid hormones. Both T_3 and T_4 enter the target cell membrane by passive diffusion (and also by active uptake), but T_4 is immediately converted to the more active T_3 and inactive *reverse* T_3 forms. Unlike the steroid hormones (c.f. Figure 3.5), T_3 enters the cell nucleus *directly* via a nuclear transport process (and an additional process involving a cytosolic thyroid hormone binding protein [CTBP]), and reacts with specific thyroid hormone receptors (TRs), already bound to target DNA regulatory elements; a nuclear protein TRAP (thyroid hormone receptor auxiliary protein) is required for efficient binding of TRs to DNA. The consequent increase (or decrease) in synthesis of specific proteins, mediates the thyroid hormone 'response' of the target cell. T_3 can also interact directly with mitochondria to increase energy production.

cell nucleus with a resultant stimulation (or repression) of target gene expression. Translocation of T_3 into the nucleus also involves a direct active uptake mechanism, together with an additional process involving a low affinity *cytosolic thyroid hormone binding protein (CTBP)* (Figure 4.4; see also Chapter 3, p. 30). In contrast with steroids however, the formation of the T_3-receptor complex occurs *directly* at the nuclear level, since the unliganded TRs are already bound to regulatory *thyroid hormone response elements (TREs)* on the target DNA even in the absence of thyroid hormone. After synthesis, TRs are not, therefore, retained in the cytoplasm in combination with heat shock proteins; a *thyroid hormone receptor auxiliary protein (TRAP)* however, appears to be important for stabilization of TR binding to the nuclear DNA within the cell. Several isoforms of the TR protein ($TR_{\alpha 1-3}$, $_{\beta 1-2}$) have been identified, with characteristically different tissue distributions (e.g. $TR_{\beta 2}$ is only expressed in the pituitary); the biological functions of all these variants have not, however, been clearly established. Some evidence for more rapid non-nuclear effects of thyroid hormones, mediated by surface membrane receptors has also been adduced.

Clinical Disorders

Apart from *diabetes mellitus*, thyroid dysfunction is one of the most common endocrine disorders encountered in adults, affecting up to 10% of the UK population (females are generally more prone to thyroid disorders than males). The two most common thyroid diseases are inadequate thyroid function, *hypothyroidism*, and excessive thyroid function, *hyperthyroidism (thyrotoxicosis)*.

Thyroid Hyposecretion

ADULT HYPOTHYROIDISM

Hypothyroidism can develop as a result of a functional defect in the thyroid itself (*primary hypothyroidism*) or as a consequence of reduced stimulatory input from the pituitary (*secondary hypothyroidism*). Primary hypothyroidism is most commonly caused by an autoimmune destruction of the thyroid gland, leading to a deficiency in the amounts of circulating thyroid hormones (*Hashimoto's thyroditis*). The condition is typically slow to develop, has a strong familial tendency and is most prevalent in middle-aged women, although it may also occur in men at any age. It is characterized by the appearance of destructive serum antibodies to thyroglobulin and to cytoplasmic components of the thyroid follicular cells (microsomal peroxidase enzyme), and a progressive infiltration of the gland by lymphocytes and plasma cells. A painful diffuse swelling of the gland (*goitre*) may be present in the early stages of the disease.

> ☞ *Goitre* is the name given to any enlargement of the thyroid that may be associated with decreased, normal or increased thyroid activity. Any substance (natural or otherwise) that can induce one is called a *goitrogen* (e.g. **goitrin**, present in cabbages, turnips or cauliflower). *Lithium carbonate*, used in the treatment of manic depression, is a potential goitrogen due to its ability to interfere with thyroid hormone release.

The main symptoms of primary hypothyroidism include:

1. *Low BMR* — a general slow-down of bodily processes, slow movements and reflexes, muscle cramps.
2. *Weight gain* and *cold intolerance* (impaired calorigenesis), decreased sweating, constipation, menstrual disturbances (heavy periods).
3. *Myxoedema* — characteristic skin changes; the skin of both the hands and face thickens and becomes coarse, dry and puffy, due to subcutaneous deposition of semi-fluid mucopolysaccharide material; hair loss.
4. *Tiredness/lethargy* — weakness, slowness of thought, memory impairment, depression, slow, hoarse speech, bradycardia.
5. *Increase in plasma carotene concentration*, producing a yellowish, jaundice-like tinge to the skin [the low levels of thyroid hormone impede the normal synthesis of vitamin A from carotenes in the liver, which then accumulate in the blood].
6. *Serum T_3/T_4 levels are low*, but TSH levels are *high* due to a lack of negative feedback effects. Abnormally high levels of plasma cholesterol may also be present.

> ☞ Total (bound + free) circulating T_3 and T_4 in the serum can be measured by sensitive radioimmunoassay (RIA) procedures. These values can be influenced by changes in the concentration of thyroid hormone binding proteins (e.g. during pregnancy, oestrogen therapy or severe illness). An accurate immunoradiometric assay (IRMA) for serum TSH, utilising highly specific monoclonal TSH antibodies is also available. Measurements of free T_3/T_4 can also be made using RIA kits or more cumbersome equilibrium dialysis methods.

Treatment. Thyroid hormone replacement therapy is necessary for life; this is administered in the form of **thyroxine sodium** tablets (*Eltroxin;* 50 μg daily initially, rising to 100–200 μg daily), or **liothyronine sodium (T_3)** (*Tertroxin;* 20 μg tablets every 8 hours or by slow intravenous injection), which has a more rapid onset of action, useful in cases of severe hypothyroidism (myxoedema coma with hypothermia). Frequent measurements of serum TSH are made to check for adequacy of the replacement therapy; patients also need to be advised on the importance of taking the thyroid hormone replacements on a regular basis. Maintenance doses of thyroid hormone may need to be increased during pregnancy.

Childhood (Congenital) Hypothyroidism

Uncorrected hypothyroidism at birth (usually due to ectopic location or failure of proper development of the thyroid) leads to *cretinism*; infant subjects are dwarfed, with a protruding tongue and abdomen, mentally retarded, and have coarse scanty hair and dry, yellowish skin. Early diagnosis is essential (based on TSH assay of a heel-prick blood sample absorbed onto filter paper), followed by thyroxine replacement therapy (10 μg/kg up to 50 μg daily).

Development of primary hypothyroidism in early childhood, *(juvenile hypothyroidism)*, is usually characterized by stunted growth, delayed sexual development and mental slowness, usually reflected by poor performance at school. The replacement dose of thyroxine (25–200 μg daily) needs to be carefully adjusted to ensure that catch-up growth progresses at a normal rate.

Some other important causes of hypothyroidism include:

1. *Surgical removal (partial thyroidectomy)* or *radioactive iodine (^{131}I)* treatment of thyroid tissue for the relief of *hyper*thyroidism.

2. *Inadequate TSH production* due to pituitary or hypothalamic disease; this rare *secondary* condition is not normally accompanied by a goitre or myxoedema, but is associated with deficiencies in the other pituitary trophic hormones, and is therefore treated with a combination of glucocorticoid/sex steroid and (later) thyroid hormone replacement therapy.

3. *Iodine deficiency: endemic goitre* may result from a low dietary intake of iodide (e.g. from seafood); this is pretty rare in Western countries where iodized table salt is generally available, but may still occur in certain parts of the world that are distant from the sea, or in mountainous regions.

4. *Amiodarone administration:* the iodine-containing cardiac anti-arrhythmic agent **amiodarone** (*Cordarone X*) can interfere with the peripheral conversion of T_4 to T_3, leading to an increase in serum T_4 (and inactive rT_3) levels; significant clinical symptoms of hypothyroidism (or even *hyper*thyroidism: see below) may develop in some patients taking this drug, that usually reverse within a few weeks following drug withdrawal. The drug is not therefore recommended for use in patients with a history of thyroid disease.

Thyroid Hypersecretion

Hyperthyroidism (thyrotoxicosis) is most commonly caused by an overactivity of the thyroid gland itself resulting from an autoimmune condition known as *Graves' disease*. The serum of such patients contains specific *thyroid-stimulating immunoglobulins (TSIs)* that bind to the TSH receptors on the follicular cells, and like natural TSH, *stimulate* the cells to produce thyroid hormone. Antithyroglobulin and antimicrosomal autoantibodies may also be present. The disease is 5–8 times more prevalent in 40–50 year old females than in males, and is commonly associated with other autoimmune disorders such as *myasthenia gravis, Addison's disease*, and *pernicious anaemia*.

The major symptoms of Graves' disease are:

1. *High BMR* — a general acceleration of body metabolism; increased heat production leading to *heat intolerance, excessive sweating* and *warm skin*.

2. *Weight loss* (despite a good appetite), due to muscle wasting (*thyrotoxic myopathy*); diarrhoea; menstrual disturbances.

3. *Rapid pulse, tremor, palpitations* and other tachycardias (atrial fibrillation in the elderly), hypertension: [the increased thyroid hormone secretion generally exaggerates responses of the sympathetic nervous system due to an increase in the number and affinity of β-adrenoceptors].

4. *Restlessness*, overanxiety, nervousness, irritability, hyperexcitability and emotional instability.

5. *Eye changes** — possible eyelid retraction and protrusion of the eyeballs (*exophthalmos* or *proptosis*) in about 50% of patients, due to thickening of the extraocular muscles caused by lymphocyte infiltration and deposition of mucopolysaccharide and oedema around the orbital soft tissues.

6. *Diffuse toxic goitre* (symmetrical swelling of the thyroid).

7. *Serum T_3/T_4 levels are raised*, but the serum TSH level is *low* (undetectable) due to excessive negative feedback effects of the elevated T_3/T_4 hormones on the anterior pituitary.

☞ The development of Graves' ophthalmopathy cannot be directly attributed to the excess levels of T_3/T_4, and may even occur in patients in the absence of other hyperthyroid symptoms. In extreme cases, ocular pain with blurring or loss of vision, and corneal ulceration may occur. Like Graves' disease, it is thought to be due to an autoimmune process directed against the orbital connective tissue or muscle cells, although the nature of the autoantibodies involved and the factors involved in their induction are not known. Achievement of normal hormone levels by therapy of hyperthyroidism is important in reducing the long-term persistence of the condition. Systemic administration of glucocorticoids, surgical therapy or orbital irradiation (sparing the lens and retina) can also be effective in the treatment of local eye symptoms in severe cases.

TREATMENT

There are three methods currently available for the treatment of Graves' hyperthyroidism: *antithyroid drugs, radioactive iodine (^{131}I) or surgery.*

Antithyroid Drugs.

1. *Thiourea derivatives (thionamides)*: **Carbimazole** (*Neo-Mercazole*) or **propylthiouracil**. These agents are accumulated by the thyroid, and reduce thyroid hormone secretion by diverting oxidized iodide away from the *thyroid peroxidase* enzyme involved in the production and coupling of iodotyrosines within the gland. Carbimazole may also have some specific immunosuppressant effects on the thyroid. They are used mainly for the long-term treatment of hyperthyroid patients and also for the preparation of patients prior to radioiodine treatment or subtotal thyroidectomy. Carbimazole is rapidly converted to an active metabolite **methimazole** in the body (only the latter drug is used in the USA). Unlike carbimazole, propylthiouracil can inhibit the de-iodination of T_4 to T_3 in peripheral tissues. In an attempt to induce a lasting remission, carbimazole/methimazole therapy is usually started with a relatively large daily dose (20–60 mg) for 4–8 weeks, then progressively reduced to a maintenance dosage continued for up to 12–18 months, followed by gradual withdrawal. Retreatment may, however, be necessary 1–2 years after stopping therapy (a major disadvantage of these drugs). Although T_3/T_4 synthesis is rapidly inhibited, the clinical response to carbimazole or propylthiouracil can be delayed for 1–2 weeks until the endogenous stores of thyroid hormone become depleted. Overtreatment with antithyroid drugs may even lead to symptoms of *hypo*thyroidism developing in some patients.

   A recently introduced 'block-and-replace' treatment protocol using daily doses of carbimazole (40–60 mg) together with replacement doses of thyroxine (50–150 μg daily) for up to 18 months, has been found to produce significantly lower relapse rates in thyrotoxic patients.

   Side effects associated with *carbimazole* or *propylthiouracil* include *severe skin rashes, nausea, vomiting* and (rarely) *agranulocytosis* (a low white blood cell count), heralded by a *severe sore throat, mouth ulcerations* and *fever* requiring immediate withdrawal of the drug and treatment with antibiotics. Propylthiouracil (at tenfold higher dosage; 300–600 mg daily) may then be substituted in patients unable to tolerate carbimazole and *vice versa*. Carbimazole and propylthiouracil may be given during pregnancy and breast-feeding, provided the smallest possible effective doses are used and foetal development is closely monitored throughout.

2. *Aqueous iodine solution BP (Lugol's iodine)*: A solution of 5% iodine dissolved in 10% potassium iodide in purified water, is usually given orally (5–10 drops diluted with milk or water, three times daily) to hyperthyroid patients for about 10–14 days prior to thyroid surgery, in order to reduce the size and vascularity of the gland. Under such conditions *excess* iodine (converted to iodide in the liver) transiently inhibits thyroid hormone production by an unknown mechanism (this effect is usually absent in normal, euthyroid individuals); Lugol's solution is of no use in the long-term control of hyperthyroidism, since the antithyroid effects of the iodine do not persist for more than a few weeks, but it can be of value in the emergency treatment of *thyrotoxic crisis* (see below) where a rapid relief of symptoms is required.

   ☞ *Potassium iodide tablets* (60 mg twice daily) may also be given for 7–10 days prior to operation, and contain sufficient iodine to suppress thyroid function.

3. β-*Adrenoceptor blockers*: Non-cardioselective beta-blockers such as **propranolol** (*Inderal*), **nadolol** (*Corgard*) or **sotalol** (*Beta-cardone)* may be administered initially along with antithyroid medication to rapidly ameliorate the tachycardia, palpitations, agitation and tremor symptoms of hyperthyroidism. They have no effect on thyroid hormone secretion, and are therefore of little use in long-term management of thyrotoxicosis.

Radioactive Iodine. Iodine-131 (^{131}I), given as a tasteless solution of Na^{131}I is often the treatment of choice for thyrotoxic patients over 40 years and for the elderly. *It is absolutely contraindicated for use in pregnant women (due to risk of foetal hypothyroidism) or in very young children.* Radioactive iodine acts by accumulating in the thyroid and selectively destroying the overactive thyroid tissue by local irradiation (mainly β, with some γ emission) over a period of 1–6 months. During this lag period, symptoms may be treated with carbimazole or propranolol. Patients must be adequately controlled into a 'euthyroid' state with antithyroid drugs prior to giving ^{131}I. Drugs are usually stopped two days before and following radiotherapy to permit optimal thyroidal ^{131}I uptake.

Side effects: initial discomfort in the neck and transient worsening of symptoms may occur for a few days after treatment (*radiation thyroditis*). Undertreatment may allow the condition to persist, and even adequate therapy may eventually result in the development of *hypo*thyroidism over several years. Regular measurements of serum TSH levels are therefore essential during the post-treatment period. Repeated treatment may be necessary in some persistently hyperthyroid patients after 6–9 months.

Surgery. Partial thyroidectomy offers prompt and effective control (particularly in patients with recurrent hyperthyroidism after drugs), but is a technically demanding procedure even for a skilled surgeon, since the *parathyroid glands* and *recurrent laryngeal nerves* may also be inadvertently damaged (resulting in hypoparathyroidism and voice changes respectively). As with radioiodine treatment, problems may arise later from resultant *hypo*thyroidism. Prior to surgery, it is common practice to give antithyroid drug (and β-adrenoceptor blocker) therapy in order to restore the patient to a 'euthyroid' metabolic state, followed by aqueous iodine solution to reduce the vascularity of the gland (making it easier and safer to operate).

☞ In recent years, there has been a significant shift in therapeutic preference towards radioactive iodine therapy (rather than antithyroid drugs or surgery) for the treatment of hyperthyroidism.

OTHER COMMON CAUSES OF HYPERTHYROIDISM

Toxic Multinodular Goitre. This is quite common in elderly patients, and is due to the development of multiple hyperactive thyroid nodules. The patient may have normal thyroid hormone levels initially, but eventually the nodules function independently, and mild hyperthyroidism develops, without exophthalmos. Usual treatment is with surgery or radioactive iodine since relapses are common after a course of antithyroid drugs. The underlying cause of the condition is unknown.

Solitary Toxic Nodule. This can occur in patients at any age, due to the development of a single overactive thyroid nodule (e.g. a benign autonomous follicular adenoma, not under pituitary control), that secretes excess thyroid hormones. Patients present with mild symptoms of hyperthyroidism and may be treated with radioiodine or partial thyroidectomy.

Subacute (De Quervain's) Thyroiditis. This is a rather uncommon, self-limiting inflammatory condition of the thyroid, most likely of viral origin, that can follow an upper respiratory tract infection. Swelling and tenderness of the thyroid may be present, with pain on swallowing, depending on the severity of the inflammation. Some symptoms of hyperthyroidism e.g. weight loss, excessive sweating, irritability, tachycardia and tremor may also occur due to inflammatory release of preformed thyroid hormone. Treatment is with oral analgesics and corticosteroids for thyroid pain and inflammation, and propranolol for hyperthyroid cardiac effects. A transient phase of mild *hypo*thyroidism, may follow the condition.

Thyrotoxic Crisis ('Thyroid Storm'). This is a rare, though serious medical emergency that can occur due to a sudden release of large amounts of thyroid hormone in an otherwise controlled hyperthyroid patient following sudden stress or infection, or after surgery/radioiodine therapy in unprepared patients. Extreme restlessness, confusion, abdominal pain, tachycardia (with possible heart failure) and fever are present. Immediate treatment is begun with propranolol (slow intravenous infusion), antithyroid drugs and aqueous iodine (orally or by nasogastric tube if necessary) together with corticosteroids, antibiotics and intravenous maintenance fluids/electrolytes. The hyperthermia may be treated with ice packs.

Secondary hyperthyroidism may also arise from the following:

1. Surreptitious (secret) ingestion of excessive amounts of thyroid hormone in an attempt to lose weight (*Thyrotoxicosis factitia*).
2. TSH-producing pituitary adenoma (rare).
3. Ovarian teratoma with thyroid elements (*Struma ovarii*).
4. Metastatic thyroid carcinoma (follicular type).
5. Treatment with the cardiac anti-arrhythmic drug **amiodarone** (*Cordarone X*).

☞ The *TRH test* can be useful in the diagnosis of hyperthyroidism. A 400 μg dose of TRH is injected intravenously and plasma levels of TSH are measured before and 20–30 minutes after injection, to test for an adequate anterior pituitary response. In primary hyperthyroid patients, the expected rise in plasma TSH (generally between 5–30 mU/l) is suppressed due to the ongoing negative feedback inhibition of the pituitary by the high thyroid hormone levels. In some patients, TRH injection can cause a brief rise in blood pressure, tachycardia or bronchospasm.

'Sick Euthyroid' Syndrome

In addition to the conditions of hypo- and hyperthyroidism described above, abnormal results of the thyroid function tests can be encountered in patients suffering from various acute or chronic illnesses or stresses. These conditions include: *myocardial infarction, renal failure, cirrhosis, serious burns, sepsis, surgical trauma, anorexia,* and *malnutrition.* Abnormally low serum T_3/T_4, with high levels of reverse T_3 levels can result from altered rates of peripheral conversion of T_4 to T_3 and/or reverse T_3, or from changes in TBG levels. Basal serum TSH levels are generally *normal* in these patients, which may serve as an important diagnostic feature of the 'sick euthyroid' syndrome. Treatment of the underlying disorders eventually leads to a normalization of the affected indices of thyroid function. ■

Review Questions

Question 1: State the location of the thyroid gland and explain briefly, its histological structure.

Question 2: Name the hormones secreted by the thyroid and describe how they are stored within the gland.

Question 3: What is the function of the parafollicular C cells?

Question 4: Name the amino acid from which thyroid hormones are derived.

Question 5: Describe how thyroid follicular cells are capable of accumulating iodide from the blood.

Question 6: Outline the use of radioactive pertechnetate in diagnostic scanning.

Question 7: Describe the mechanisms controlling thyroid hormone release.

Question 8: Explain how thyroid hormones are transported in the bloodstream.

Question 9: What do the abbreviations T_3, T_4 and rT_3 represent? Which is the more active hormone?

Question 10: Summarize the main effects of thyroid hormone on:
    (a) calorigenesis
    (b) carbohydrate/fat/protein metabolism
    (c) maturation of the CNS
    (d) skeletal growth and maturation.

Question 11: Outline how T_3 and T_4 exert their biological effects via intracellular receptors.

Question 12: Describe the causes, symptoms and treatment of:
    (a) adult hypothyroidism
    (b) congenital and juvenile hypothyroidism.

Question 13: Define the meaning of the term goitre; what is a goitrogen.

Question 14: What type of drug is amiodarone? Why is this agent not recommended for use in patients with a history of thyroid disease?

Question 15: List the major symptoms of hyperthyroidism (thyrotoxicosis: Graves' disease).

Question 16: Explain the three methods used for treating Graves' hyperthyroidism and state their limitations.

Question 17: Explain the rationale for use of Lugol's iodine and β-adrenoceptor blockers in the treatment of thyrotoxicosis.

Question 18: Describe some other common causes of hyperthyroidism.

Question 19: What is the TRH test? How may it be used in the diagnosis of hyperthyroidism?

Question 20: Explain the causes of 'sick euthyroid' syndrome.

Clinical Case Studies

Patient 1

A 33 year old female was seen by her GP, complaining of nervousness, increased sweating, palpitations, weakness, weight loss (despite a good appetite) and amenorrhoea of three month duration. She had lost about eight kg (18 lb) weight since the appearance of symptoms about one year ago. The patient had no prior medical history, but there was a strong family history of thyroid disease. She was referred to a hospital Endocrinology Department for further investigation. Clinical examination revealed a very anxious, restless young female of slender build. She had fine tremors, and her palms were warm and moist. Despite it being winter, she was wearing only light clothing, and claimed that she did not feel cold. Her heart rate was 116 beats/min and blood pressure was 140/80 mmHg. The thyroid gland was diffusely enlarged, and there was a mild protrusion of her eyes. Cardiac examination showed a soft systolic murmur, best heard in the pulmonary area. Pulmonary examination was unremarkable, as was the rest of the examination.

Thyroid function tests revealed an elevated serum T_4 of 16.8 µg/dl (normal: 4–12 µg/dl) and TSH < 0.05 µU/ml (normal 0.5–5 µU/ml). Total serum T_3 was 369 ng/dl (normal 80–180 ng/dl) and TSH receptor antibodies were strongly positive.

Question 1: *What is the patient most likely to be suffering from?*
Question 2: *What is the recommended treatment for her condition?*
Question 3: *What other possible treatments are there, and what are their side effects?*

Answer 1: This patient has classic signs of *autoimmune thyroid disease (Graves' disease) with hyperthyroidism.* It is the most common cause of hyperthyroidism, more commonly seen in females than in males, and often associated with other autoimmune disorders. The diagnosis is verified by the laboratory findings showing elevated levels of serum T_3/T_4 with a very low level of TSH (due to negative feedback effects of excessive thyroid hormone). The presence of TSH receptor antibodies (*thyroid-stimulating immunoglobulins (TSIs)*) that continuously stimulate thyroid hormogenesis, confirms the autoimmune nature of the disease. The major symptoms of Graves' disease include: excessive sweating, warm skin and weight loss, due to a general acceleration of body metabolism with increased heat production, and tachycardia, tremor and palpitations, due to general overactivity of the sympathetic nervous system. Cardiac murmur, commonly found in hyperthyroidism, can be attributed to an increased cardiac output. Protrusion of the eyeballs (*exophthalmos*) is also seen in ca. 50% of hyperthyroid patients, due to lymphocyte infiltration and fluid deposition around the orbital soft tissues.

Answer 2: Following diagnosis of Graves' disease, the patient was treated with an antithyroid drug (*propylthiouracil, 450 mg daily*) and a β-adrenoceptor blocker (*propranolol, 80 mg daily*), becoming asymptomatic in 3 weeks. She refused to be treated with radioactive iodine, and was therefore continued on propylthiouracil; her thyroid indices normalized in 16 weeks.

Answer 3: Treatment for Graves' disease includes medical therapy with antithyroid drugs (thionamides) (together with beta-blockers), radioactive iodine (^{131}I) thyroid ablation, or surgical subtotal thyroidectomy. Beta-blockers are useful for the short-term treatment of the tachycardia, palpitations, nervousness and tremor symptoms, while long-term (12–18 month) treatment with thionamides is aimed at controlling the excessive hormone secretion. Side effects associated with propylthiouracil include skin rashes, nausea and agranulocytosis. With medical treatment alone, about 50% of patients remain in remission after completion of treatment. The recovery from exophthalmos is unpredictable. Use of radioactive iodine is based on its selective accumulation in the thyroid gland, and consequent destruction of overactive thyroid tissue by local irradiation. A possible side-effect of such radiotherapy is the higher risk of developing *hypothyroidism* (ca. 50% over 10 years) compared to medical or surgical treatments. Radioactive iodine cannot be used in patients who are pregnant or in very young children.

Patient 2

A 77 year old woman was admitted to hospital for evaluation of rectal bleeding. The patient was noticed to be lethargic and complained about the hospital air conditioning being too cold. She was unable to elaborate on any previous medical illnesses, and had not seen a doctor for several years.

Clinical examination revealed a puffy face with some periorbital oedema, cool dry yellowish skin, slow heart rate (58 beats/min), loss of eyebrows and non-pitting oedema. Her temperature was 35°C, blood pressure was 150/90 mmHg, and deep tendon reflexes showed a delayed relaxation phase. Her thyroid gland was firm and non-tender. She also complained of some weight-gain over the past year, difficulty in 'remembering things', always feeling tired (particularly in the evenings) and being constipated.

Laboratory tests revealed a normal full blood count (FBC) and urinalysis, but blood chemistry showed an elevated cholesterol level of 13.8 mmol/l (268 mg/dl). Thyroid function tests showed a serum TSH of 102 μU/ml and a total T_4 of 0.9 μg/dl.

Question 1:   *What is the likely diagnosis and cause of this patient's condition?*
Question 2:   *How would her condition be treated, and what special considerations need to be applied in her case?*

Answer 1:   This is a typical case of *primary hypothyroidism*, where symptoms have been neglected for a long time (commonly mistaken for normal aging). Major manifestations of hypothyroidism include: easy fatigability, mental slowness and memory impairment, weight gain, constipation, cold intolerance (due to impaired heat production), muscle cramps, slow heart rate (bradycardia), hair loss, dry skin, puffy face (due to *myxoedema*), husky voice and slow relaxation of deep tendon reflexes. Reduced conversion of plasma carotenes to vitamin A in the liver may give a yellowish colour to the skin. A rise in blood cholesterol level may also occur due to a decrease in its rate of degradation. Hypothyroidism is diagnosed by documentation of low serum thyroxine (T_4) levels with high levels of TSH in suspected individuals.

Idiopathic atrophic thyroid disease is the most common cause of hypothyroidism in the elderly, and is presumably the end stage of a destructive autoimmune thyroid disease, causing a deficiency in circulating thyroid hormone. When the thyroid gland itself is dysfunctional, the term *primary hypothyroidism* is used, whereupon low serum T_3/T_4 levels and high TSH levels would be expected (due to lack of negative feedback effect). The condition is typically slow to develop, as in this patient. When the defect lies in the pituitary or hypothalamus, the condition is known as *secondary hypothyroidism*, and would be characterized by low serum levels of *both* TSH and T_3/T_4.

Answer 2:   On diagnosis of primary hypothyroidism, the patient was started on *liothyronine sodium (T_3), 20 μg daily*, with 20 μg dose increments made every five weeks, till TSH and thyroxine levels stabilized. Starting replacement treatment with small doses is important in the elderly, to avoid precipitating ischaemic cardiac episodes (anginal pain). Drugs that interfere with the absorption of liothyronine from the gut (e.g. diphenylhydantoin, activated charcoal or cholestyramine [anion-exchange resin]) are also to be avoided. This patient became completely asymptomatic in six months, and was able to take daily walks and watch late night television — something she could never do before.

UK/USA Drugs — Trade names		
	UK	**USA**
Thyroid hormones L-thyroxine sodium	Eltroxin	Levothroid/Levoxine Levoxyl/Synthroid
Liothyronine sodium	Tertroxin	Cytomel Triostat
Antithyroid drugs Carbimazole Methimazole*	Neo-Mercazole	Tapazole
Propylthiouracil		Propylthiouracil
β-adrenoceptor blockers Propranolol	Inderal	Inderal Inderide
Nadolol	Corgard	Corgard Corzide
Sotalol	Beta-cardone	Betapace

*Methimazole is an active metabolite of carbimazole. Carbimazole is converted to methimazole *in vivo*.

References

Books

- **Cawson RA, McCracken AW, Marcus PB, Zaatari GS.** (1989). Diseases of the endocrine system. In *Pathology. The mechanisms of disease*, 2nd ed. CV Mosby Co, 434–460
- **Chandrasoma P, Taylor CR.** (1991). The thyroid gland. In *Concise Pathology*, 1st ed. Prentice-Hall, USA, pp. 839–855.
- **Dong BJ.** (1975). Diseases of the thyroid. In *Applied Therapeutics for Clinical Pharmacists*, edited by MA Koda-Kimble, BS Katcher, LY Young, 2nd ed. Applied Therapeutics Inc, San Francisco, pp. 494–529
- **Farwell AP, Braverman LE.** (1996). Thyroid and antithyroid drugs. In *Goodman & Gilman's The Pharmacological Basis of Therapeutics*, edited by JG Hardman, LE Limbird, A Goodman, Gilman *et al*, 9th ed. McGraw-Hill, USA, pp. 1383–1409
- **Fletcher RF.** (1987). Thyroid. In *Lecture Notes on Endocrinology*, 4th ed, Blackwell Scientific Publications, Oxford, pp. 68–98
- **Genuth SM.** (1993). The thyroid gland. In *Physiology*, edited by RM Berne, MN Levy, 3rd ed. Mosby-Year Book Inc, USA, pp. 932–948
- **Goodman HM.** (1988). Thyroid gland. In *Basic Medical Endocrinology*, Raven Press, New York, pp. 45–70
- **Greenspan FS.** (1994). The thyroid gland. In *Basic & Clinical Endocrinology*, edited by FS Greenspan, JD Baxter, 4th ed. Appleton & Lange, Connecticut, pp. 160–226
- **Griffin JE.** (1988). The thyroid. In *Textbook of Endocrine Physiology*, edited by JE Griffin, SR Ojeda. Oxford University Press, New York, pp. 222–244
- **Guyton AC, Hall JE.** (1996). The thyroid metabolic hormones. In *Textbook of Medical Physiology*, 9th ed. WB Saunders Company, USA, pp. 945–956
- **Hedge GA, Colby HD, Goodman RL.** (1987). Thyroid physiology. In *Clinical Endocrine Physiology*. WB. Saunders Co, Philadelphia, pp. 101–126
- **Hershman JM.** (1988). Thyroid disease. In *Endocrine Pathophysiology: a patient orientated approach*, 3rd ed. Lea & Febiger, Philadelphia, pp. 37–76
- **Junqueira LC, Carneiro J, Long JA.** (1986). Adrenals & other endocrine glands. In *Basic Histology*, 5th ed. Lange Medical Publications, Connecticut, pp. 446–467
- **Laurence DR, Bennett PN.** (1992). Endocrinology III: thyroid hormones, antithyroid drugs. In *Clinical Pharmacology*. Churchill Livingstone, pp. 581–589
- **Marshall WJ.** (1988). The thyroid gland. In *Illustrated Textbook of Clinical Chemistry*. Gower Medical Publishing, pp. 139–154
- **Safrit HF.** (1992). Thyroid disorders. In *Handbook of Clinical Endocrinology*, edited by PA Fitzgerald, 2nd ed. Prentice-Hall, USA, pp. 156–226

Journal Articles

- **Beswick T.** (1988). Thyroid disorders and their treatment. *The Pharmaceutical Journal*, April 9th, 470–472
- **Burch HB, Wartofsky L.** (1993). Graves' ophthalmopathy: current concepts regarding pathogenesis and management. *Endocrine Rev*, 14, 747–793
- **Carter JA, Utiger RD.** (1992). The ophthalmopathy of Graves' disease. *Annu Rev Med*, 43, 487–495
- **Cheung EN.** (1985). Thyroid hormone action: determination of hormone-receptor interaction using structural analogs and molecular modelling. *Trends in Pharmacol Sci*, 6, 31–34
- **Clark J.** (1996). A guide to management of thyroid disorders. *Prescriber*, 7(18), 55–64
- **Edmonds C.** (1991). Thyroid disease: diagnosis and treatment options. *Prescriber*, (39), 33–36
- **Evans RM.** (1988). The steroid and thyroid hormone receptor superfamily. *Science*, 240, 889–895
- **Ichikawa K, Hashizume K.** (1995). Thyroid hormone action in the cell. *Endocrine J*, 42, 131–140
- **Lazar MA.** (1993). Thyroid hormone receptors: Multiple forms, multiple possibilities. *Endocrine Rev*, 14, 184–193
- **Lazarus JH.** (1997). Hyperthyroidism. *Lancet*, 349, 339–343
- **Nemere I, Zhou L-X, Norman AW.** (1993). Nontranscriptional effects of steroid hormones. *Receptor*, 3, 277–291
- **Wartofsky L.** (1993). Has the use of antithyroid drugs for Graves' disease become obsolete? *Thyroid*, 3, 335–344

5 Endocrine Secretions of the Pancreas

Structure and Histology

The pancreas has both exocrine and endocrine functions, carried out by distinctly different groups of cells. The endocrine portion is limited to small rounded clusters of glandular tissue, the *islets of Langerhans*, ca. 300 μm in diameter, that form <2% of the mostly *exocrine* (acinar) pancreatic mass, but nevertheless secrete two crucially important peptide hormones involved in blood glucose regulation, **insulin** and **glucagon**. There are about 10^6 islets scattered throughout the human pancreas, each constituting an independent secretory unit receiving a copious capillary blood supply via the gastroduodenal and superior mesenteric arteries, and draining ultimately through the splenic and superior mesenteric veins into the portal vein.

Histology

Each pancreatic islet consists of ca. 2,500 specialized epithelial cells embedded within the exocrine tissue; four principal types of cell have been identified using immunohistochemical or other specialized staining methods:

1. *α-cells* (ca. 20% of islet population) are the largest cell type, localized towards the outer margins of the islet, produce **glucagon**;
2. *β-cells* are smaller and more numerous (ca. 70%), occupying the central area of the islet, produce **insulin**;
3. *δ-(D) cells* (ca. 10%), distributed along the islet periphery, produce **somatostatin** (which is a hypothalamic GH release-inhibiting hormone; see Chapter 2) that may exert a localized *paracrine* action on other islet cells to influence both insulin and glucagon secretion.
4. The so-called *PP (or F) cells* constitute a minor proportion of the islet cells, and secrete **pancreatic polypeptide;** the functional role of this peptide in the release of other pancreatic hormones is not, however, fully understood.

Neighbouring islet cells are metabolically and electrically linked via *gap junctions*, perhaps ensuring a synchronized mode of hormone secretion. Sympathetic and parasympathetic nerve fibres terminate close to all types of islet cell.

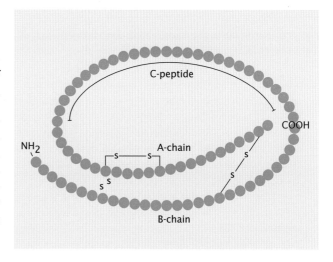

Figure 5.1. The proposed structure of the insulin precursor molecule, proinsulin. Before secretion, the C-peptide fragment connecting the A and B peptide chains of the insulin molecule is enzymatically cleaved to yield insulin. Note the two disulphide bridges connecting the peptide chains and the third intrachain link within the A chain.

Pancreatic Hormones

Insulin

BIOSYNTHESIS, STORAGE AND RELEASE

Insulin is a 51 amino acid polypeptide synthesized in the β-cells as a precursor molecule, **proinsulin** (derived from a larger insulin gene product, *preproinsulin*); the folded proinsulin structure consists of an A-chain and a B-chain, linked by two disulphide bridges, together with a 31 amino acid intermediate connecting peptide (*C-peptide*). An additional disulphide link is also present within the A-chain portion (Figure 5.1).

Following synthesis, the proinsulin is stored within cytoplasmic secretory granules (located close to the cell membrane), where the C-peptide is slowly cleaved by peptidase enzymes to yield insulin and C-peptide molecules. The insulin is retained in the core of the granule in the form of a polymeric complex in association with zinc.

Release of insulin (together with equimolar amounts of inactive C-peptide and some proinsulin) occurs by exocytosis in a Ca²⁺-dependent manner; once released into the portal circulation, the insulin is rapidly metabolized by the liver (and kidneys) with a plasma half-life of ca. 5–10 min. The detection of C-peptide in the blood (by radioimmunoassay) may be used as a measure of β-cell activity in diabetic patients (see below).

Control of Release. Insulin release is regulated by a number of stimulatory and inhibitory factors, although a basal level of secretion is normally maintained. Release is principally influenced by:

1. *The blood glucose concentration*: One of the major physiological determinants of insulin secretion by the β-cells, is the level circulating glucose in the blood; an *increase* in blood glucose level (above ca. 4.5 mmol/l) stimulates both synthesis and release of insulin by a direct feedback mechanism. Insulin release occurs in a characteristically *biphasic* manner (early and late phases) in response to continuous glucose stimulation, suggesting the existence of at least two storage pools for insulin within the cells.

    ☞ This stimulatory effect of glucose depends on its initial facilitated transport into the β-cell (via the GLUT2 carrier protein), and subsequent metabolism to yield an increase in intracellular levels of ATP. The high level of ATP then *inhibits* the activity of a special class of *ATP-sensitive K⁺ channels (K$_{ATP}$)* present in the β-cell membrane, with a resultant cell depolarization, influx of Ca²⁺ and triggering of hormone release. With normal levels of intracellular ATP, these channels remain open, and thereby maintain the β-cell in a hyperpolarized (non-secreting) state.

2. *Other islet hormones*: Glucagon and *somatostatin* may also influence insulin release indirectly (stimulation or inhibition respectively) by modulating the levels of intracellular cAMP; a rise in cAMP and subsequent activation of *protein kinase A*, generally promotes exocytosis of insulin and *vice versa* (Figure 5.2).

3. *Gastrointestinal hormones:* Several hormones released from the gastrointestinal tract (see below p. 66) e.g. *gastrin, secretin, cholecystokinin* and particularly *gastric inhibitory peptide (GIP)* (from mucosal endocrine K-cells) stimulate insulin release directly. These humoral effects may be physiologically important in dealing with a sudden surge in blood glucose following a meal. It is well known that an *orally*-administered dose of glucose releases more insulin than an intravenously administered one, indicating the important role of gastrointestinal factors (released during food ingestion) in enhancing insulin secretion.

    ☞ A *truncated glucagon-like peptide (tGLP-1* or *incretin)*, derived from a **preproglucagon** precursor molecule (see below) is secreted by endocrine L cells of the lower intestine following a meal or glucose ingestion. tGLP-1 is a potent stimulator of insulin secretion from pancreatic β-cells (insulinotropic action); the antidiabetogenic effects of tGLP-1 are currently being investigated for use in the treatment of patients with *diabetes mellitus* (see below).

4. *Amino acids and fatty acids: Arginine, leucine* and some other amino acids derived from protein digestion are potent stimulators of insulin release; these effects are generally synergistic (mutually-enhancing) with those of glucose. An increase in free fatty acid levels also promotes the secretion of insulin.

5. *Some other hormones: Growth hormone (GH), glucocorticoids and thyroid hormone* may stimulate insulin release indirectly by increasing the blood glucose level.

6. *The autonomic nervous system:* Parasympathetic (vagal) nerve stimulation increases insulin secretion while the *dominant* effect of sympathetic nerve stimulation is to *inhibit* release; the latter is due to activation of α-adrenoceptors on the β-cell membrane, leading to a *decrease* in intracellular levels of cAMP (Figure 5.2) (activation of β-adrenoceptors by adrenergic agonists has the opposite effect).

PRINCIPAL ACTIONS OF INSULIN

Insulin is the only hormone with the ability to directly *lower* the blood glucose level. It may generally be regarded as an *anabolic* hormone, promoting the storage of chemical energy derived from food in the form of *glycogen, proteins* and *lipids (triglycerides), while suppressing the mobilization (catabolism) of stored nutrients*; the major target organs for insulin action are consequently the liver, muscles and adipose tissue, i.e. organs that are specialized for energy storage. Some tissues of the body such as kidney, brain, or red blood cells are less sensitive or unresponsive to this hormone.

The two principal types of effect of insulin on target cells may be summarized as follows:

1. *Effects on solute transport*: an *increase* in the cellular transport of glucose, amino acids and fatty acids;
2. *Modulation of key intracellular metabolic pathways*: an *increase* in the synthesis of glycogen, proteins and fats and *an increase* in the synthesis of nucleic acids by direct stimulation of DNA and RNA formation.

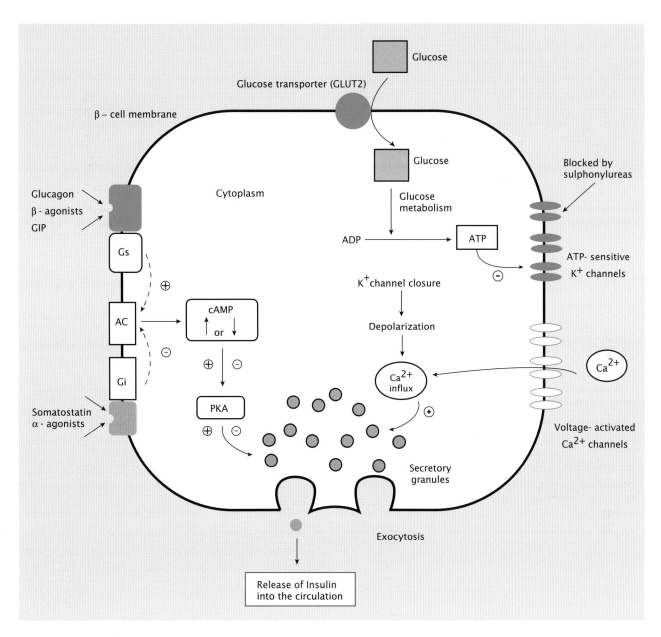

Figure 5.2. Mechanisms involved in the control of insulin release by the pancreatic β-cell. External glucose is transported into the cell via a specific carrier protein (GLUT2) and metabolised to produce a rise in intracellular ATP. The increased level of ATP then *closes* ATP-sensitive K+ channels with a resultant depolarization of the cell, influx of Ca²⁺ through voltage-sensitive Ca²⁺ channels and release of insulin from secretory granules. Release is also modulated by other factors operating via surface receptors linked to adenylate cyclase (AC) and cAMP production.
Note: specific block of ATP-sensitive K+ channels by *antidiabetic sulphonylurea drugs*, may also induce release.

Carbohydrate Metabolism: Effects on Glucose Transport. Plasma glucose is normally maintained within the range of 3.6–6.4 mmol/l (65–115 mg/dl); however, for tissues such as *skeletal and cardiac muscle* and *adipose cells*, glucose cannot penetrate the cell membrane by simple (or facilitated) diffusion down its concentration gradient, and intracellular glucose is consequently very low. In the presence of insulin, glucose uptake by these tissues is rapidly increased, due to the selective mobilization (and activation) of preformed glucose transporter molecules (GLUT4) from intracellular vesicles to the cell membrane. This process is believed to be mediated by an insulin-dependent phosphorylation of proteins involved in vesicle translocation (Table 5.1).

↑ in glucose transport in muscle and fat	
↑ in muscle amino acid uptake	
↑ in protein synthesis	↓ in muscle protein breakdown
↑ in fat synthesis in liver and adipose tissue (lipogenesis)	↓ in fat breakdown in adipose tissue (lipolysis)
↑ in conversion of glucose to glucose-6-P in liver ↑ in glucose metabolism (glycolysis)	↓ in liver gluconeogenesis (synthesis of glucose from non-carbohydrate sources e.g. amino acids, lactate and glycerol)
↑ in glycogen synthesis in liver and muscle (glycogenesis)	↓ in glycogen breakdown (glycogenolysis)

Table 5.1. Major metabolic effects of insulin.

Some tissues (e.g. liver, red blood cells and particularly brain cells) depend on facilitated diffusion only (via specific glucose transporter proteins) for glucose entry, therefore an adequate blood glucose level is essential for their normal function. Proximal tubule cells of the kidney and luminal epithelial cells of the small intestine also possess an *active* Na^+-dependent glucose transporter (SGLT1) that is independent of insulin.

☞ At least five structurally related, facilitative glucose transporter proteins (termed GLUT1–5) have so far been identified, each with a characteristic tissue distribution; only the GLUT4 isoform however (uniquely expressed in skeletal muscle, cardiac muscle and fat cells), is regulatable by insulin.

Carbohydrate Metabolism: Effects on Metabolic Pathways. Insulin also has numerous and complex effects on the intracellular pathways involved in *glucose* and *glycogen* metabolism.

The principal effects of insulin are:

1. *Stimulation* of glycogen synthesis in skeletal muscle, liver and adipose tissue by a direct *increase* in *glycogen synthase* and a *decrease* in *glycogen phosphorylase* activity.
2. *Increase* in hepatic glucose phosphorylation (due to *stimulation* of *glucokinase* activity), and a *decrease* in glucose dephosphorylation (due to *inhibition* of *glucose-6-phosphatase* activity).
3. *Increase* in glucose metabolism (*glycolysis*) with a simultaneous *decrease* in liver *gluconeogenesis*. Key enzymes involved in glycolysis (conversion of glucose into pyruvate

and lactate) including *6-phosphofructokinase* and *pyruvate kinase* are stimulated by insulin, whereas those required for gluconeogenesis (formation of glucose from amino acids, lactate and glycerol) including *pyruvate carboxylase* and *phosphoenolpyruvate carboxykinase* are inhibited.

The general decrease of glucose entry into the blood from hepatic glycogen stores, along with the increase in cellular glucose uptake, accounts for the unique blood glucose-lowering effect of insulin in the body. The major pathways for glucose and glycogen metabolism affected by insulin are summarized in Figure 5.3.

Protein Metabolism. Insulin stimulates the cellular active transport of plasma amino acids into muscle (thereby lowering blood amino acid levels) and also stimulates muscle protein synthesis directly, (anabolic action) while depressing protein breakdown. The lower levels of circulating amino acids contribute towards the overall decrease in liver gluconeogenesis.

Fat Metabolism. Insulin stimulates uptake of glucose into adipose cells and promotes the synthesis (*lipogenesis*) and storage of fatty acids in the form of triglycerides in both adipose and hepatic tissues (the activity of the blood capillary enzyme *lipoprotein lipase*, that facilitates the clearance of dietary fat from the plasma, is increased by insulin). It also prevents fat breakdown (*lipolysis*) by inhibiting *hormone-sensitive lipase* activity in adipose cells; the levels of circulating free fatty acids are therefore reduced (an important feature that prevents the generation of plasma *ketone bodies* (see below)). The major effects of insulin on carbohydrate, protein and fat metabolism are listed in Table 5.1.

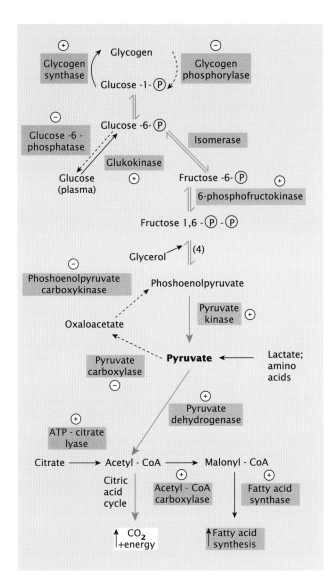

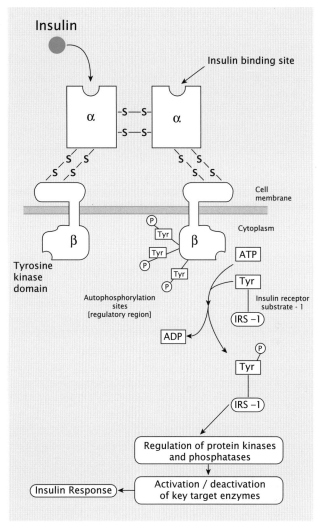

Figure 5.3. Effects of insulin on glucose, glycogen and fatty acid metabolism in the liver. Some key enzymes that are either stimulated (+) or inhibited (−) by insulin action are indicated. Insulin generally facilitates glucose oxidation (to pyruvate) and the reactions leading to glycogen and fatty acid synthesis, while inhibiting the production of glucose from amino acids, lactate and glycerol (gluconeogenesis). (Some intermediate reaction steps have been omitted for clarity.)

Figure 5.4. Cellular mechanism of action of insulin. Binding of the hormone to one external α subunit of the insulin receptor causes a conformational change, leading to autophosphorylation of three tyrosine residues on the adjacent β subunit and stimulation of intrinsic tyrosine kinase activity. Tyrosine phosphorylation of the principal insulin receptor substrate (IRS-1) enables it to act as an intermediate signalling molecule leading ultimately to activation/deactivation of key metabolic enzymes involved in mediating the insulin 'response'.

MECHANISM OF ACTION OF INSULIN

Insulin has a complex catalogue of effects on many tissues. These effects are now known to be mediated via an interaction with specific insulin receptors on the target cell surface. The insulin receptor is a large transmembrane glycoprotein (molecular mass ca. 400 kDa) composed of two identical α-subunits, each coupled to each other and to two identical β-subunits by disulphide bridges (Figure 5.4). The α-subunits, containing the high affinity insulin binding sites, are located externally, whereas the β-subunits span the cell membrane and possess an intrinsic *tyrosine-specific protein kinase* activity that is regulated by insulin binding. This kinase activity appears essential for mediating most of the metabolic actions of insulin. Some rare genetic disorders characterized by a cellular resistance to insulin (see below) are believed to result from a fault in insulin receptor structure and function.

☞ *Protein kinase* enzymes catalyse the transfer of phosphate groupings from ATP to amino acid residues on proteins, whereas *phosphatase* enzymes catalyse the hydrolytic removal of phosphate groups and therefore effectively reverse the regulatory effects of the kinases.

Following binding of insulin to one of the α-subunits, the internal β-subunit domain of the adjacent αβ dimer becomes rapidly phosphorylated (*autophosphorylation* via ATP) which in turn stimulates the intrinsic tyrosine kinase activity of the receptor. The principal intermediate cytoplasmic protein substrate for the insulin receptor kinase is termed the **insulin receptor substrate-1 (IRS-1)**, a 185 kDa peptide containing multiple potential tyrosine phosphorylation sites within its molecule. The phosphorylated sites in IRS-1 associate with high affinity with distinct cellular signalling proteins (e.g. *phosphatidylinositol-3'-kinase*) containing *Src homology 2 domains* (SH2 proteins) that ultimately mediate the multi-faceted insulin response (Figure 5.4). IRS-1 itself has no intrinsic catalytic function, but it acts as a multisite 'docking' protein that interacts with various regulatory elements during insulin signal transmission. Some key enzymes and proteins that undergo phosphorylation (via *kinases*) or dephosphorylation (via *phosphatases*) in response to insulin are listed in Table 5.2.

☞ The receptor for the **insulin-like growth factor (IGF-1**; see Chapter 2) shares many structural similarities with the insulin receptor, and also utilizes the IRS-1 signalling pathway.

Prolonged stimulation of the insulin receptor leads to internalization (endocytosis) of the insulin-receptor complex and insulin degradation, that may serve to terminate the insulin signal; (various *phosphatases* may also be involved in the reversal of insulin effects). Some of the internalized receptors are degraded, while most are recycled to the plasma membrane. The internalized insulin receptor can still function as a tyrosine kinase, suggesting a supplementary role in the signal transduction process. Many features of the insulin action pathway however e.g. the mechanism by which insulin influences DNA and RNA synthesis, are still relatively unclear.

Glucagon

Glucagon is a simple, 29 amino acid unbranched peptide that is synthesized in pancreatic islet α-cells from a larger

Enzymes undergoing *dephosphorylation*	Effect on enzyme activity
Glycogen synthase	Activation
Pyruvate dehydrogenase	Activation
*Acetyl-CoA carboxylase	Activation
Glycogen phosphorylase	Inactivation
Phosphorylase kinase	Inactivation
Hormone-sensitive lipase	Inactivation

Enzymes and proteins undergoing phosphorylation	Effect
cAMP phosphodiesterase	Activation
ATP-citrate lyase	Activation
§Protein phosphatase-1G (PP1G)	Activation
Proteins controlling intracellular translocation of glucose transporter molecules	Transfer of glucose transporters (GLUT4) from intracellular stores to plasma membrane

* The involvement of insulin in the dephosphorylation/ phosphorylation of this enzyme is still controversial.

§ Insulin is known to activate *protein phosphatase-1G (PP1G)*, involved in the dephosphorylation of *glycogen synthase* (and phosphorylase kinase), by means of a phosphorylation reaction on the G-subunit (site 1); this is mediated by an *insulin-stimulated protein kinase (ISPK)*.

Table 5.2. Some key enzymes that are *dephosphorylated* (via protein phosphatases) or phosphorylated (via kinases) in response to insulin.

preproglucagon precursor molecule and stored in the form of cytoplasmic granules. Unlike insulin, its structure is identical in different mammalian species. It is released from the islet cells (into the portal circulation) by a process of Ca²⁺-dependent exocytosis, mediated by a rise in the level of intracellular cAMP (c.f. mechanism of insulin secretion; Figure 5.2). Once released, it is rapidly metabolized by the liver and kidney (plasma half-life ca. 3–5 min). **Gut glucagon** is also secreted by specialized α-like cells in the mucosa of the stomach and duodenum, and has the same actions as the pancreatic hormone.

CONTROL OF RELEASE

Glucagon release is affected by the following factors:

1. *The blood glucose concentration:* In contrast to insulin, an *increase* in blood glucose level (e.g. following a meal) *inhibits* glucagon release and vice versa.

   ☞ The sensitivity of islet α-cells to glucose is dependent on an adequate level of insulin. Thus, under conditions of insulin deficiency (i.e. *diabetes mellitus*; see below), the normal secretion of glucagon in response to a lowered blood glucose may be impaired.

2. *Other islet hormones:* Glucagon release is *inhibited* by both *somatostatin* and *by insulin*; (note that insulin release is directly *stimulated* by glucagon).
3. *Gastrointestinal hormones: cholecystokinin, gastrin* and *gastric inhibitory peptide (GIP)* stimulate glucagon release.
4. *Amino acids and fatty acids:* Certain amino acids, particularly *arginine* and *alanine* stimulate glucagon secretion, whereas increased levels of free fatty acids cause an *inhibition* of its release (cf. opposite effect of fatty acids on insulin release). The increased secretion of glucagon in response to a protein-rich meal enables the liver to dispose of the excess plasma amino acids by gluconeogenesis.
5. *The autonomic nervous system:* Both sympathetic and parasympathetic nerve stimulation increase the secretion of glucagon. Secretion is also enhanced by stressful stimuli (e.g. vigorous exercise) most likely acting via the sympathetic nervous system.

ACTIONS OF GLUCAGON

The main actions of glucagon are generally *opposite* to those of insulin, and tend to protect the body from hypoglycaemia (blood glucose <2.8 mmol/l). It is a *catabolic* hormone that *raises* the blood glucose concentration by affecting carbohydrate, protein and fat metabolism in the liver, its major target organ. These effects are mediated by specific membrane glucagon receptors (coupled to adenylate cyclase) that generate an increase in intracellular cAMP levels in the target cells.

The principal actions of glucagon may be summarized as follows:

1. *Increase in hepatic glycogenolysis* and *gluconeogenesis,* leading to an increase in production and release of glucose into the blood.
2. *Increase in lipolysis* and mobilization of fatty acids (from triglycerides), resulting in increased levels of circulating *ketoacids,* acetoacetate and β-hydroxybutyrate (*ketogenesis;* see below). This effect is mediated by an increase in *hormone-sensitive lipase* activity (via elevation of cAMP).

INSULIN-GLUCAGON MOLAR RATIO

Compared to insulin, the basal level of glucagon secretion is relatively high; the intake of food however, induces a greater relative change in the level of plasma insulin than plasma glucagon. The so-called *insulin-glucagon ratio* (normally around 2.0) may thus vary considerably in response to the availability of nutrients and the immediate energy requirements of the body: e.g. the ratio may be decreased to <0.5 during periods of fasting or after a prolonged period of exercise (due to preferential release of glucagon); under these conditions, glycogenolysis and gluconeogenesis are promoted in order to provide an adequate blood glucose level (particularly for the central nervous system) and lipolysis is facilitated to provide fatty acids and ketones as energy sources for oxidation by muscle and liver. When nutrients are abundant (e.g. after a mixed meal), the ratio can rise to ca. 10 or more due to increased insulin release, thereby promoting the deposition of glycogen, proteins and fat.

Other Islet β-cell Peptides

AMYLIN

Amylin (or *islet amyloid polypeptide: IAPP*) is a 37 amino acid peptide produced by the pancreatic β-cells and normally co-secreted along with insulin at very low levels (ca. 1:100 molar ratio), following nutrient stimuli. Structurally, it belongs to the **calcitonin** family of peptides, which includes calcitonin itself and the *calcitonin gene-related peptides (CGRPα and CGRPβ)* (ca. 50% homology), considered to be important regulatory neuropeptides, both in the central and peripheral nervous systems. Not surprisingly, amylin has similar (though less potent) hypocalcaemic and vasodilator effects to those of calcitonin or CGRP respectively, mediated via a specific type of G-protein coupled cell membrane receptor. Amylin can also influence carbohydrate metabolism by reducing the synthesis of glycogen from glucose in skeletal muscle, while increasing muscle glycogen breakdown to lactate (opposite actions to insulin), thereby increasing plasma lactate (and subsequently glucose) concentration; it may also exert an autocrine inhibitory effect on islet insulin secretion.

The main interest in amylin centres on its recently proposed role in the aetiology of *type II, non-insulin-dependent diabetes mellitus (NIDDM; see below):* plasma amylin levels are generally found to be *high* in patients with chronic NIDDM, and low or deficient in *type I, insulin-dependent diabetics (IDDM).* When present in excess, amylin can aggregate to form insoluble pancreatic *amyloid* fibrils which are deposited within the islet cells, and may be a critical factor contributing to their eventual degeneration; [this effect of pancreatic amylin is reminiscent of that of the *amyloid β-peptide (Aβ)* which forms neurotoxic amyloid fibrils in the brains of subjects with Alzheimer's disease].

Since amylin functionally opposes the metabolic effects of insulin on skeletal muscle, its excess production has also been suggested as a possible cause of insulin resistance, glucose intolerance and obesity associated with type II diabetes. Therapeutic strategies aimed at inhibiting pancreatic amyloid production or blocking peripheral amylin action are currently being investigated for possible use in the treatment of NIDDM.

PANCREASTATIN

Pancreastatin (PST) is a 49 amino acid peptide, derived from *chromogranin A (CgA)*, an acidic glycoprotein that is co-secreted with catecholamines from sympathetic nerve terminals and adrenal chromaffin cells. Since CgA is processed to PST in the plasma, it has been suggested that the blood levels of this peptide may reflect excessive sympathetic nerve activity in essential hypertension. Circulating plasma PST-like immunoreactivity may also be used as a useful clinical marker of certain tumours of the sympathetic nervous system (*neuroblastomas, ganglioneuromas*) and also the pituitary (*adenomas*), pancreas and gut, which are known to release significant amounts of this (and other) *regulatory peptides*[*]. Within the pancreas, PST is co-released with insulin, and can inhibit both insulin and glucagon secretion, as well as exocrine pancreatic secretions. PST is also present in the gut (stomach, duodenum, small intestine and colon) and is stored and co-secreted along with **parathyroid hormone (PTH)** in the parathyroid gland (see Chapter 7); its functional role at these sites, however is unclear.

*Endocrine secretions of the gastrointestinal tract
A large variety of peptide hormones are also secreted by specialized enteroendocrine cells of the gastrointestinal mucosa to affect gastrointestinal secretion and motility [the entire study of endocrinology is, in fact, founded on the discovery of the first gut hormone — **secretin**, by Bayliss & Starling in 1902]. These gut peptides have common structural and functional characteristics and can be grouped into hormone 'families', each group presumably arising from a common ancestral gene; not all these substances however, have a known physiological function.
Some principal examples include:
The gastrin family: *gastrin, cholecystokinin (CCK)*

The secretin family: *secretin, glucagon, vasointestinal polypeptide (VIP), gastric inhibitory peptide (GIP)*

The pancreatic polypeptide family: *pancreatic polypeptide (PP), peptide YY (PYY), neuropeptide Y (NPY)*

The tachykinin family: *substance P, gastrin-releasing peptide (GRP)*

Orphan peptide family: *motilin, neurotensin, somatostatin, galanin, pancreastatin*

Some of the peptides, derived from the gut (and pancreas) circulate in the bloodstream to affect distant organs, and may therefore be regarded as true hormones in the classical endocrine sense (e.g. gastrin, CCK, GIP, secretin); others serve a *paracrine* or *autocrine* role, being secreted in a more localized manner to affect nearby (or the same) cells within the gastrointestinal system (*regulatory peptides*). Some serve a peptidergic neurotransmitter role within the enteric nervous system of the gut (e.g. VIP).

A large number of gut peptides are also localized in the central nervous system (and vice versa), where they are believed to act as neurotransmitters or neuromodulators (*neurocrine* role) (e.g. somatostatin, substance P, CCK). Apart from **somatostatin** and its analogue **octreotide** however, (see Chapter 2), the use of gastrointestinal peptide hormones or their antagonists in treating clinical disorders is not firmly established at present. [For a detailed description of the properties and known functions of the major regulatory peptides of the gut, see Mulvihill & Debas (1994). Nevertheless, certain gastrointestinal hormones have pathophysiological significance:

Some recognised clinical implications involving gastrointestinal peptides include:

The Zollinger-Ellison syndrome, a rare condition in which unregulated ectopic secretion of **gastrin** occurs from a gastrin-producing tumour (*gastrinoma* — usually in the endocrine pancreas or duodenum) resulting in *hypergastrinaemia*, occurrence of severe recurrent peptic ulcers (non-responsive to therapy) and unexplained diarrhoea; treatment usually consists of surgical tumour resection (where possible) or long-term therapy with a proton pump inhibitor (*omeprazole, lansoprazole*) or histamine H_2 receptor antagonist (*cimetidine, ranitidine, famotidine*).

Gastrin is secreted by endocrine G-cells of the gastric antral mucosa and also by cells of the duodenum; it is mainly responsible for stimulating acid (HCl) secretion from the gastric parietal cells, and also promoting their growth (*trophic* effect). It exists in three active forms with different peptide chain lengths (17, 34 and 14 amino acid residues). Gastrin has also been found to stimulate the growth of gastric and colorectal cancer cells; gastrin receptor antagonists are therefore being evaluated for possible therapeutic use in treating gastrin-responsive gastrointestinal cancers as well as preventing gastric ulcer formation.

Likewise, the **gastrin-releasing peptide (GRP)** is thought to act as an autocrine growth factor involved in the initiation and progression of some human breast cancers; synthetic antagonists acting at the GRP receptor may then have a possible therapeutic use in inhibiting the growth of such tumours. The measurement of certain gastrointestinal peptides in the blood by radioimmunoassay (e.g. *gastrin, VIP, glucagon, somatostatin, neurotensin*) may have a more general diagnostic value in the early detection of neuro-endocrine gastrointestinal and pancreatic tumours.

The Verner-Morrison Syndrome is a condition in which ectopic secretion of **vasointestinal peptide (VIP)** occurs from a pancreatic islet cell tumour ('*VIPoma*'; see also Chapter 2) causing a characteristic voluminous watery diarrhoea (due to overstimulation of the intestinal epithelium), hypo-kalaemia and metabolic acidosis (due to faecal loss of K^+ and HCO_3^-); specific VIP receptor antagonists may thus prove useful in the management of this condition (usually treated by surgical excision of the tumour, or subtotal pancreatectomy). It has been suggested that VIP or its analogues could also be effective, in the treatment of bronchial asthma.

VIP is a basic 28 amino acid peptide secreted mainly by enteric peptidergic nerve cells (and also pancreatic D cells) but not gut endocrine cells; its main function is to stimulate intestinal electrolyte (and water) secretion and also to relax intestinal sphincters.

Clinical Disorders

Glucagon Hyposecretion

Clinical conditions of glucagon undersecretion are not well known, although some cases of *neonatal hypoglycaemia* have been attributed to glucagon deficiency. On rare occasions, excess secretion of glucagon by pancreatic glucagon-secreting tumours (*glucagonomas*) may be encountered, and may lead to mild diabetic symptoms (e.g. hyperglycaemia and weight loss); treatment is usually by surgical removal of the tumour. **Glucagon hydrochloride** (1 mg, by intra-muscular, intravenous or subcutaneous injection) may be used clinically in the emergency treatment of severe hypoglycaemia.

Insulin Deficiency

*Hypo*secretion of insulin by the pancreas results in the common condition of *diabetes mellitus*, which affects ca. 2% of the UK population at any age. The overall prevalence of diabetes in the US is similar, with considerable ethnic differences, including a greater than 40% incidence in the Pima Indians of Arizona. It is a serious condition in which the normal conversion of glucose into energy by the body is disrupted, along with a severe reduction in the ability to store glycogen, fat and proteins; this may result in:

1. Chronic *hyperglycaemia* and *glycosuria* (high blood and urine glucose levels respectively),
2. *Polyuria* (increased urine production) with dehydration and excessive thirst (*polydipsia*),
3. *Polyphagia* (increased appetite) due to inadequate transport of glucose into cells and consequent triggering of the hunger sensation and,
4. *Wasting of muscle and fat*, with an increase in ketoacid metabolites in the blood (*ketosis*).

MAJOR CONSEQUENCES OF INSULIN DEFICIENCY

Hyperglycaemia and Glycosuria. In the absence of insulin, the blood glucose concentration (normally between 3.6–6.7 mmol/l after fasting) can rise above 35 mmol/l. Normally, glucose is filtered by the renal glomeruli, then completely reabsorbed in the kidney tubules by carrier mechanisms. However, when the filtered load exceeds the renal threshold of ca. 10 mmol/l (180 mg/dl), glucose appears in the urine and acts as an *osmotic diuretic* (retaining water in the tubules), leading to *polyuria*, dehydration and *polydipsia*. The renal threshold for glucose generally tends to increase with age. In severe cases, a profound fall in blood volume with eventual coma/death may result.

Ketosis. In the absence of insulin, *lipolysis* is stimulated, and free fatty acid levels in the blood *increase*. Fatty acids are normally converted in the liver to their intermediate *acyl CoA* derivatives, and then oxidized in the mitochondria to *acetyl CoA*; the latter enters the *citric acid cycle* to undergo further oxidation, yielding CO_2 and energy (Figure 5.5). Lack of insulin causes excess acetyl CoA to accumulate in the liver, where it condenses to form *ketone bodies: acetoacetate, 3-hydroxybutyrate* and *acetone*, which then appear in the blood (*ketonaemia*) and urine (*ketonuria*) of uncontrolled insulin-dependent diabetics; the acetone imparts a characteristic sweet smell to the breath of such patients. High concentration of ketone bodies in the circulation also induces *nausea, vomiting, metabolic acidosis (abnormally low blood pH) and ultimately a diabetic coma.*

Muscle Wasting. Insulin deficiency will tend to reduce all *anabolic* processes and facilitate *catabolic* processes; protein breakdown will therefore be increased, and blood amino acid levels will rise. This protein depletion (together with the enhanced fat breakdown) contributes to the severe muscle wasting, weakness and loss of weight found in chronic diabetics.

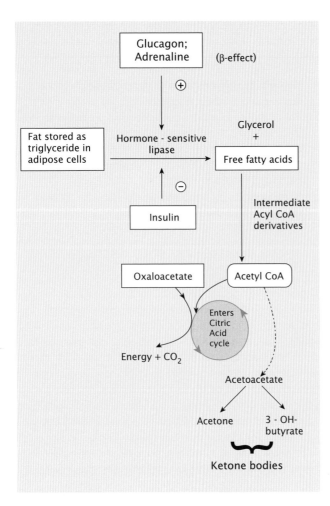

Figure 5.5. Summary of reactions involved in fatty acid metabolism (lipolysis). In the absence of insulin (as in diabetes mellitus), the inhibitory effect on the hormone-sensitive lipase activity is removed, allowing fat breakdown to predominate and free fatty acid levels in the blood to increase. Under such conditions, accumulation of acetyl CoA in the liver leads to formation of *ketone bodies*.

Secondary Diabetes

Hyperglycaemia may also be caused by an *excess* secretion of various hormones including **cortisol, adrenaline, growth hormone, glucagon** and **thyroxine**, all of which may therefore induce a *secondary diabetes*. The condition may also be caused by administration of certain drugs that reduce glucose tolerance (e.g. *thiazide diuretics*) or influence carbohydrate metabolism (e.g. *oestrogen-containing oral contraceptives* and *corticosteroids*).

Primary Diabetes Mellitus

This may be classified into two types, based on the patient's requirement for insulin therapy:

INSULIN-DEPENDENT DIABETES MELLITUS (IDDM; TYPE I)

This accounts for ca. 10–20% of all diabetic cases. It is usually acute in onset, and occurs mainly in young non-obese individuals during childhood or at puberty (although adults at any age may also be affected). The condition is characterized by a selective destruction of the pancreatic islet β-cells, such that *very little or no insulin production is present*; such patients therefore require regular insulin injections for treatment. Subjects with IDDM also commonly possess *serum antibodies directed against their islet β-cells (islet cell antibodies; ICAs)*, or much less frequently, against insulin itself or the insulin receptors. These autoimmune antibodies can be detected months or even several years before main clinical features develop, and may therefore be useful as a diagnostic marker in susceptible individuals (i.e. first degree relatives of known type I diabetics).

☞ The incidence of other autoimmune diseases e.g. Addison's disease, thyroid disease and pernicious anaemia is markedly increased in patients with IDDM. Although IDDM is not directly inheritable, patients that possess certain *human leucocyte antigen (HLA) types* carry an increased risk of developing this disease that may be inherited. The HLA antigens are cell-surface glycoproteins that are present on all cell-types except red blood cells and sperm; they form part of a set of cell-surface molecules determined by the so-called *major histocompatibility complex (MHC)* of genes present on the short arm of human chromosome 6. The six important HLA gene loci (termed A, B, C, DP, DQ and DR) code for over 100 possible known types of HLA antigen, with each individual possessing a fixed combination of these molecules. The particular antigens that predispose a person towards IDDM are HLA-DR3, DR4 (or both) and DQw8 (*w* indicates a provisional identification); (interestingly, the presence of HLA-DR2 somehow *protects* against the development of diabetes). Some other autoimmune diseases have also been linked to particular HLA groupings (e.g. Graves' disease and HLA-B8).

It has been suggested that the development of certain specific HLA antigens may increase the susceptibility of islet β-cells to viral attack (e.g. by mumps, rubella or coxsackie B4 virus) or to damage by environmental toxins, so that an abnormal autoimmune response ultimately develops against altered self-antigens presented on the β-cell membrane.

NON-INSULIN-DEPENDENT DIABETES MELLITUS (NIDDM; TYPE II)

This type of diabetes (formerly called *maturity-onset diabetes*) is the more common (80–90% of all cases) and is normally slower to develop, usually in older (over 40 years) more obese individuals; it is claimed to affect ca. 5% of the world population. Such patients *continue to secrete some insulin*, therefore insulin therapy is usually not required; however the amount secreted is generally not sufficient to maintain a normal blood glucose level. Some patients may, in fact, show a characteristic *insulin resistance* (coupled with a *high* blood insulin level or *hyperinsulinaemia*, leading eventually to β-cell exhaustion) suggesting a defect in the action of insulin (particularly in stimulating muscle glucose uptake) at the receptor or postreceptor levels. The insulin resistance leads to an increase in the rate of lipolysis and elevation in free fatty acid levels; this, coupled with an increased liver glucose production and reduced glucose uptake, results in a significant hyperglycaemia. Despite the above abnormalities, the development of *ketosis* in type II diabetes is relatively rare.

☞ The exact origin of this insulin resistance in NIDDM remains controversial, although it is clear that a direct relationship exists between the degree of obesity of an individual and the resistance to insulin action. A defect in insulin receptor function due to a genetic mutation of the insulin receptor gene, may be one principal mechanism involved. Other possibilities include the synthesis of structurally abnormal insulins, the presence of a defect in the *glucokinase* enzyme gene, or a specific down-regulation of the insulin-sensitive glucose transporter protein (GLUT4) in target tissues, following sustained hyperglycaemia.

Unlike type I diabetes, there is *no HLA link or presence of autoimmune ICAs*, however a very strong genetic component exists in the development of NIDDM (more significant than with type I); this means there is a significant probability of inheriting the disease from a type II diabetic parent. Moreover, if one identical twin develops type II diabetes, there is an increased probability that the other twin will also develop it.

A missense mutation in the glucagon receptor gene has recently been shown to be highly associated with the development of type II diabetes.

Gestational Diabetes

This condition may develop during pregnancy (2–3% of cases) and resolve after delivery. It can however, recur during subsequent pregnancies, or develop later in life, into type II diabetes unrelated to pregnancy (ca. 50% risk). Good control of maternal blood glucose during pregnancy is important, as it improves the general outcome for the foetus (reducing risk of major congenital abnormalities or foetal death); the babies of diabetic mothers however, still tend to be larger than normal for their gestational age (*macrosomia*), and may suffer from the *respiratory distress syndrome* (due to lack of lung phospholipid surfactant). Gestational diabetes may be treated by controlled diet alone,

or by administration of insulin (the insulin requirement may progressively increase during the pregnancy); oral hypoglycaemic drugs (see below) are not generally recommended to be taken while pregnant, due to an increased risk of congenital abnormalities or development of neonatal hypoglycaemia. Established type II diabetics may need to switch to insulin therapy during pregnancy.

Some Late Clinical Features of Diabetes

MACROVASCULAR COMPLICATIONS

All chronic diabetics (i.e those that have had the condition for 20 years or more) have a high risk of developing serious cardiovascular disease (atherosclerosis) at an earlier age than other people; this is partly due to the derangement of lipid and cholesterol metabolism (causing *hyperlipidaemia*, and *hypercholesterolaemia*). The larger blood vessels e.g. coronary and cerebral arteries, as well as peripheral vessels become more prone to occlusion (thrombosis), leading to possible ischaemic heart disease (myocardial infarction), or stroke. Limb ischaemia, ultimately requiring amputation of a foot or a leg for gangrene is also more likely.

MICROVASCULAR COMPLICATIONS

Long-term diabetic patients (particularly those with a poor history of glycaemic control) also have an increased risk of developing damage to *small* blood vessels (*microangiopathy*). This involves a thickening of the basement membrane (associated with an increased protein glycosylation) and increased permeability of the fine capillaries, particularly in the *eye* and *kidney*, resulting in retinal damage (*retinopathy*) and defective kidney filtration (*nephropathy*) with appearance of protein in the urine (*proteinurea*). Diabetes still remains the most common cause of blindness in middle-aged adults; cataract formation (increased lens opacity), particularly in young diabetics, and refractive changes in the lens are also common. Frequent ophthalmic observation of diabetics is therefore considered essential.

Microvascular damage to blood vessels in the skin may cause skin lesions (*dermopathy*), particularly in the feet, where poor circulation (coupled with a general delay of tissue healing and increased susceptibility to infection) can result in *foot ulceration* and even *gangrene of the toes*. Diabetics (particularly the elderly) are thus advised to wear comfortable shoes, to avoid cutting their own toe-nails and to undergo regular foot examination by a chiropodist.

PERIPHERAL NEUROPATHY

Peripheral nervous tissue (mainly sensory nerves), can become progressively damaged, leading to pain and eventual numbness in the feet; foot ulceration and infection may therefore occur without the patient being aware of the problem. Common early signs of diabetic neuropathy include the loss of deep tendon reflexes and vibration sense in the lower limbs. Damage to sympathetic and parasympathetic nerves (*autonomic neuropathy*) may also result in the loss of cardiovascular reflexes.

☞ Both neuropathy and cataract formation in diabetics has been associated with the intracellular accumulation of *sorbitol* within the peripheral nerve or lens tissue; this nondiffusible sugar is formed in excess when glucose levels are high (catalysed by the enzyme *aldose reductase*), and may then induce osmotic swelling and damage in certain vulnerable cells.

Insulin Excess

Hypersecretion of insulin (*hyperinsulinism*) can either result from a rare insulin-secreting (usually benign) tumour of the pancreatic islets (*insulinoma*) or very rarely from a diffuse proliferation of endocrine cells within the pancreas (*islet β-cell hyperplasia*; more common in children). The excess insulin action leads to a chronic intractable hypoglycaemia (associated with fasting or exercise), manifested mainly as episodic neurologic symptoms (*neuroglycopenia*) e.g. lack of concentration, confusion, disorientation, amnesia, abnormal behaviour (often misdiagnosed as psychiatric illness), and possible seizures or coma.

Treatment of insulinomas is usually by surgical removal of the tumour(s), although these may be very small and difficult to locate. Alternative medical therapy involves long-term oral administration of **diazoxide** (*Eudemine*), a potent inhibitor of pancreatic insulin secretion. Diazoxide is used to normalize blood glucose levels prior to tumour surgery, and in the management of β-cell hyperplasia; it is also a powerful directly-acting vasodilator, and may be given by rapid intravenous bolus (300 mg) to lower blood pressure quickly in cases of acute hypertensive emergency. Blind subtotal resection of the pancreas (pancreatectomy) is less favoured as a mode of treatment.

Diagnosis and Monitoring of Diabetes

URINE GLUCOSE TESTS

An initial simple test for monitoring of urinary glucose (not necessarily diagnostic of diabetes) may be made using plastic, glucose-sensitive reagent strips (e.g. *Clinistix, Diabur-Test* or *Diastix*; *Tes-Tape* in the USA); these provide a colour reaction proportional to the urine glucose concentration, which may be compared visually with a colour chart. Alternatively, diagnostic reagent tablets (*Clinitest*; poisonous: not to be taken!), which rely on the standard reduction by

glucose, of an alkaline copper solution, may also be used for simple screening purposes (less popular). Urinalysis is a less accurate method of assessing diabetic control than direct blood glucose monitoring.

☞ Diagnostic tablets (*Acetest*) or ketone-sensitive reagent strips (*Ketostix* or *Ketur Test*) for *ketone* (mainly acetone and acetoacetic acid) detection in the urine, are also available, as are tests for urinary proteins (albumin) (using *Albustix* or *Albym-Test* reagent strips); the latter test is considered useful for the early detection of *diabetic nephropathy* (see below).

BLOOD GLUCOSE TESTS

Self measurement of glucose in a blood drop (usually obtained by pricking the side of a finger) may also be made using specific glucose-sensitive colour test strips (containing *glucose oxidase*) that are either read visually against a colour chart (e.g. *Dextrostix*; *Glucose VT*) or used in conjunction with a portable reflectance meter (e.g. the pocket *Accutrend Mini* or *Accutrend Alpha* with *BM-Accutest* strips or *Reflolux S* meter, with *BM-Test* 1–44 strips: *Boehringer Mannheim Diagnostics*) (Figure 5.6). In the USA, the *One Touch* (*Lifescan*) blood glucose monitoring system is widely used.

Although somewhat expensive, such meters can provide a rapid and reliable measurement of blood glucose within the range of ca. 0.5–30 mmol/l and are therefore ideally suited for the maintenance of accurate home monitoring records. Patients, however, need to be carefully advised on the correct methods for obtaining the blood (several spring-loaded lancet pens are available; e.g. *Softclix; Boehringer Mannheim*) and for recording and interpreting the results.

A postprandial (after food) blood glucose level of between 4–10 mmol/l is considered as an optimal target for a controlled diabetic.

GLYCOSYLATED HAEMOGLOBIN (HbA$_{1C}$)

Dipstick tests are useful for providing immediate information about a patient's degree of diabetic control; however, in order to obtain an assessment of more long-term glycaemic control over a preceding period of about four weeks, a laboratory measurement of *glycosylated haemoglobin* levels (also called *glycated haemoglobin* or *HbA$_{1C}$*) in the blood, can be made using chromatographic, electrophoretic or radioimmunoassay techniques. The slow chemical (nonenzymatic) reaction between glucose and haemoglobin yields a small glycosylated fraction (termed HbA$_{1C}$), normally comprising ca. 4–6% of the total blood haemoglobin. Other circulatory proteins (e.g. albumin, fructosamine) or structural proteins (e.g. collagen, myelin and lens crystallins) can also become glycosylated. A close linear correlation exists between the %HbA$_{1C}$ level and the mean blood glucose concentra-

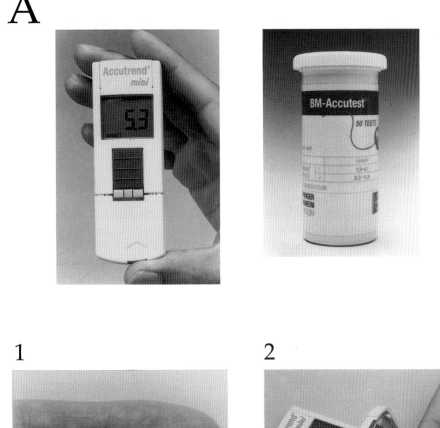

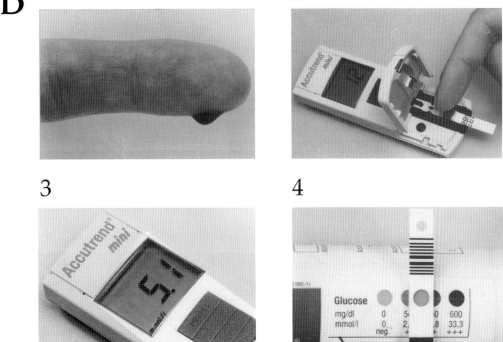

Figure 5.6. Measurement of blood glucose by means of a glucose-sensitive test strip and portable reflectance meter.
A. Example of a commercially available 'pocket' glucose meter (*Accutrend 'mini'*) that can provide a rapid digital reading of the blood glucose level (sensitivity range 1.67–22.2 mmol/l). The meter is used in conjunction with *glucose oxidase*-impregnated test strips (*BM-Accutest*). B. The recommended procedure for obtaining a measurement involves (1) washing hands thoroughly, then obtaining a blood drop from a side finger prick; (2) the blood is soaked onto the pad of a reagent strip and placed into the meter; (3) after 12 seconds, the meter displays the blood glucose level; (4) a rough visual check can also be made against a colour scale. (Photographs kindly provided by Boehringer Mannheim UK Ltd.)

tion measured over a previous 2–3 month period in both diabetic and non-diabetic individuals, thereby enabling an estimate of chronic glucose homeostasis to be made. A glycosylation level of ca. 8.4% is to be expected for a moderately well controlled type I diabetic patient, whereas a level exceeding 10% would indicate a more strict control regimen is required. The glycosylation of lens crystallins has been implicated in the formation of diabetes-related cataracts.

☞ In the *oral glucose tolerance test (OGTT)* for diabetes, a 75 g glucose drink (usually *Lucozade*) is given to an overnight fasted patient, and estimations of venous plasma glucose are obtained at zero time and then at half-hourly intervals for 2–3 hours (while still fasting). Normally, plasma glucose should not exceed 8.5 mmol/l at any time during the test, and should return to the fasting level of ca. 4–6 mmol/l after 2 hours. In cases of *impaired glucose tolerance (IGT)*, the fasting plasma glucose level is usually normal, but remains elevated (between 7.8–11.1 mmol/l) at 2 hours after the glucose load. A diagnosis of diabetes is made if the fasting plasma glucose is above 7.8 mmol/l, a high plasma glucose level (>11.1 mmol/l) is attained at 2 hours and the rise is more prolonged.

☞ Plasma (or serum) glucose concentrations tend to be ca. 10% higher than *whole blood* glucose levels.

Treatment of Diabetes

Education and counselling of the patient about their condition and treatment is all important. It is also necessary to advise on the self-monitoring of blood/urinary glucose or ketones and the correct injection techniques for insulin administration.

The major aims of treatment are:

1. To keep blood glucose near to normal (between 4 and 10 mmol/l) over 24 hours (*particularly avoiding hypoglycaemia*), thereby minimising the risk of long-term complications. Very strict control in more elderly patients may be difficult to achieve.
2. To ensure that the patient has sufficient energy for normal work and recreation (and for steady growth in young patients).
3. To ensure the patient 'feels well', and maintains a normal body weight (*obesity should be avoided*).

This control may be achieved using a combination of three methods: *diet, insulin* or *oral hypoglycaemic (antidiabetic) drugs*, according to the type and severity of diabetes, and the body weight and occupation of the person.

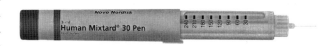

Figure 5.7. Disposable preloaded pen injector containing a pre-mixed biphasic insulin formulation (*Human Mixtard 30 Pen*). (Photographs kindly provided by Novo Nordisk Ltd, UK.)

TYPE I DIABETES

Insulin replacement therapy is required for life, coupled with frequent self-monitoring of blood/urine glucose and ketones. Insulin doses are given on an individual basis by *subcutaneous* injection, once or twice a day (before breakfast and/or before the evening meal), or more often as governed by a patient's needs (5–20 units/dose is usually sufficient). Small adjustments in dose (in 0.5–2 unit increments) can be made throughout the day, based on the pattern of the glycaemic response following each administration. If a meal is missed, an appropriate reduction in insulin dose would be required.

Insulin pens. Nowadays the use of *insulin injection 'pens'* (Figure 5.7) that can deliver metered doses of insulin from a preloaded disposable pen (*Lilly Humaject; Novo Nordisk Human Mixtard pen*) or replaceable cartridge (e.g. *NovoPens*, for use with *Novo Nordisk Penfill* cartridges; [*Novolin Pen* in the USA]) offers a reliable and more convenient alternative to the injection of insulin via a conventional plastic syringe; such pens (although more costly) are particularly advantageous for use by partially sighted or more elderly diabetic patients that would normally experience some difficulty in drawing up their daily doses.

It is recommended that injection sites are rotated frequently (outer thighs, upper arms, lower abdomen or buttocks) in order to avoid skin hardening or development of local skin reactions e.g. fat atrophy (*lipodystrophy*; now less common with human or highly purified animal insulins) or *fat hypertrophy*.

☞ Formulations of insulin combined with absorption enhancers (e.g. deoxycholate or laureth 9) for intranasal administration, are currently being investigated.

Insulin Pumps. Systems for delivery of a continuous subcutaneous infusion of soluble insulin (CSII) via a portable battery-operated pump have also been developed; these consist of a small external infusion pump with an insulin reservoir (ca. 3 ml), which can be programmed to provide various 'basal' rates of insulin delivery throughout the day (via an in-dwelling subcutaneous catheter), in accordance with patient self-monitoring of blood glucose levels. The pumps can also provide small bolus doses prior to each meal as needed, in an attempt to simulate the normal pattern of insulin secretion. Such 'open loop' pump therapy is most suitable for improving glycaemic control in selected type I patients with a particularly unstable diabetes; close medical follow-up is however necessary to avoid the risk of hypoglycaemia. Common complications of CSII include inflammation at the injection site, pump malfunction, catheter obstruction and systemic infection (rare). Some examples of available pumps (expensive!) include the *MiniMed 506* (MiniMed Technologies, USA) and the H-Tron V100 (Disetronic Medical Systems, Switzerland).

Implantable programmable insulin infusion pump systems (very expensive!) are currently undergoing intensive clinical trials throughout Europe; these small radio-controlled units (ca. 5 year life) are introduced subcutaneously within a skin pocket in the abdomen, with a catheter placed peritoneally. They are particularly useful in the management of type I diabetics with resistance to conventional subcutaneous or intramuscular insulin. Apart from mechanical failure of the system, pump movement and possible development of infection at the implantation site, blockage of peritoneal catheters due to insulin aggregation and precipitation at body heat can be a major problem.

So-called *'closed loop'* pump systems (artificial pancreas) consist of an external infusion pump, an automatic blood glucose sensor and a microprocessor for analysis of blood glucose data and for adjusting the rate of insulin delivery; these systems are more suitable for hospital, research or 'intensive care' environments, where critical blood glucose control is essential (e.g. during surgery or emergency treatment of diabetic ketoacidosis; see below). Several types of miniaturized glucose sensor suitable for long-term subcutaneous implantation are presently being evaluated; these mainly utilize a glucose oxidase/hydrogen peroxide amperometric detection system, designed to transmit sensor data to a remoter reservoir. Development of a local inflammatory tissue reaction to the implanted devices may however, limit their glucose sensitivity.

A novel non-invasive glucose monitoring system based on 'reverse iontophoresis' of glucose across the skin has also been described recently, but this will require further development and evaluation before becoming generally accepted.

Pancreatic islet cell transplantation. This also offers a potentially useful approach for the future treatment of diabetes. Numerous research studies conducted over the past decade have reported significant clinical improvement in glucose control in type I diabetics that received islet cells isolated from human cadavers (injected into the liver, via the portal vein) or cultured pancreatic tissue from aborted human embryos (transplanted intracerebrally). A major problem however, has been the immune rejection of the transplanted islets, which necessitates the use of ongoing (possibly damaging) immunosuppressive therapy. New methods aimed at 'hiding' islets from the host's immune system by encapsulating them within biocompatible semipermeable plastic fibres (implanted subcutaneously) are currently under investigation.

Types of Insulin Preparation. Human insulin (*Humulin; Novolin* in the USA; *Insulin lispro*) may be obtained either by modifying a precursor molecule formed by yeast cells using recombinant DNA technology (*pyr*) or biosynthetically from bacteria using recombinant DNA techniques (*prb*); [it can also be prepared by enzyme modification of pork insulin (*emp*) (B30 alanine is converted to threonine); *Human Velosulin*]. Genetically engineered human insulin is currently the treatment of choice for the majority of diabetic patients using insulin therapy. Insulins derived from porcine or bovine pancreas (the molecules vary only slightly from human insulin) are also available, but their use is progressively declining with each year. The animal insulins are prepared in highly purified form to minimize contamination by insulin derivatives and other pancreatic peptides which may be antigenic (e.g. proinsulin, C-peptide or glucagon). The use of bovine insulin is less popular, in view of its greater antigenic properties.

Solutions of soluble insulin are rapidly absorbed; therefore, to prolong their action, various insulin formulations are available in which insulin is complexed with *protamine* (a polyamine) or combined with *zinc* to form particle or crystalline suspensions which are more slowly absorbed. Mixtures of the different insulin preparations may also be used to achieve different patterns of activity. The four main types of insulin formulation used (classed according to their duration of action) along with some examples of currently available preparations are summarized in Table 5.3.

☞ Insulin in solution in pharmaceutical preparations tends to self-associate into dimers which, in the presence of zinc ions, form a stable hexameric assembly. Dimers can also exist in the plasma following insulin administration and limit the biological availability of the insulin molecule (monomer). Current research is aimed at development of *'monomeric' human insulin analogues* with less tendency to self-associate in solution, which would therefore be more rapidly absorbed following subcutaneous injection (giving an earlier postprandial hypoglycaemic response).

Unopened vials, cartridges or preloaded 'pens' containing insulin preparations should always be refrigerated (2–8°C) but *never frozen*. Vials containing a standard strength

Insulin type	Type of action	Examples	Description
Short acting	Rapid onset ($^1/_2$–1 h); peak effect at 2–4 h; duration up to ca. 8 h; useful for diabetic emergencies (i.v.)	Neutral insulin injection (B.P.) (Soluble Insulin) *Human Velosulin* *Human Actrapid* *Humulin S* *Humalog (Insulin Lispro)*	Clear buffered neutral solution
Intermediate	Slow onset (1–2 h); peak effect at 4–12 h; duration ca. 12–24 h	Isophane insulin injection (B.P.) *Human Insulatard*	Cloudy suspension of insulin-protamine complex
		Insulin zinc suspension (amorphous) (B.P.) *Semitard MC (porcine)*	Cloudy suspension of insulin-zinc complex.
		Insulin zinc suspension (mixed) *Humulin Lente*	Mixture of amorphous Zn and crystalline insulins (30/70%)
Long-acting	Delayed onset (2–4 h); peak effect at 6–12 h; duration up to ca. 36 h	Insulin zinc suspension (crystalline) (B.P.) *Human Ultratard*	Cloudy suspension of larger insulin-zinc crystalline particles
Mixtures	Biphasic action provides both rapid and prolonged effects; speed of onset depends on % of soluble insulin in mixture; duration up to ca. 24 h	Biphasic insulin injection B.P. *Rapitard MC*	Suspension of soluble and crystalline insulin (25/75%)
		Biphasic Isophane insulin B.P. *Human Mixtard 30*	Suspension of soluble and isophane insulin (variable proportions)

Table 5.3. Four main types of insulin formulation [BNF: Sept. 1996; MIMS: June 1997].

of 100 units/ml are currently available in the UK and in the USA (1 *unit* of insulin is equivalent to 0.035 mg of anhydrous insulin), along with disposable syringes calibrated in units. Insulin vials, cartridges or preloaded 'pens' in use can be kept at room temperature (up to 25°C) for up to 1 month.

TYPE II DIABETES

Since there is still some pancreatic β-cell activity in such patients, control may be possible by *diet alone*, or by use of *oral hypoglycaemic drugs* or other antidiabetic agents. However, in some type II diabetics (e.g. those showing a continued weight loss), insulin may also be required for adequate control.

Patients are advised to avoid all forms of refined sugar in their diets (e.g. jams, sweets, cakes, chocolate or sugary drinks), to restrict their intake of saturated fats or refined carbohydrates, and to increase intake of foods that have a high dietary fibre content (e.g. wholemeal bread, bran cereals and beans), since this can improve postprandial blood glucose control. Alcohol may be taken in moderation (ex-

cept in sweet wines or liqueurs), preferably followed soon after by food; it should be emphasized that alcohol itself may induce hypoglycaemia. Artificial sweeteners are also permitted. Ideally, obese patients should aim to reduce and to maintain their body weight at a more normal level; regular physical exercise is also recommended.

If an initial trial period (ca. 1–3 months) of dietary treatment alone fails to produce adequate glycaemic control, then *oral hypoglycaemic drugs* may be taken in addition. There are two types of drug that are currently used in the UK, **sulphonylureas** and **biguanides**, taken in tablet form. In the USA, the biguanide **metformin** has recently been approved for treatment of type II diabetes.

Sulphonylureas. These agents act initially to stimulate any residual capacity of the pancreatic β-cell to produce insulin owing to their specific ability to close ATP-regulated potassium channels in the β-cell membrane (see p. 60 and Figure 5.2). In the long term, they may also potentiate the action of endogenous circulating insulin on target tissues by increasing the number of insulin receptors.

Some currently used sulphonylureas include:

Tolbutamide	(*Rastinon*)
Chlorpropamide	(*Diabinese*)
Glibenclamide	(*Daonil, Euglucon*)
Glipizide	(*Glibenese, Minodiab*)
Gliclazide	(*Diamicron*)
Gliquidone	(*Glurenorm*)
Tolazamide	(*Tolanase*)

Side effects: these are very rare, but may include *skin rashes, blood disorders, fever* and *jaundice*. **Glibenclamide** appears to be the most popular, taken as a 2.5 or 5 mg tablet daily at breakfast time. **Gliclazide** and **tolbutamide** are preferred in elderly patients or those with renal impairment, because of their relatively short duration of action. **Chlorpropamide** is now rarely used in view of its particularly prolonged half-life in the body and its unusual tendency to produce *facial flushing* in some patients after drinking alcohol. Sulphonylureas may cause slight weight gain in some patients.

Biguanides. The only biguanide in current use is **metformin** (*Glucophage*), taken alone or more commonly in combination with a sulphonylurea. This drug acts primarily by stimulating muscle glucose uptake and by inhibiting both hepatic gluconeogenesis and glucose absorption from the gut. It also has some appetite-suppressant action which may be useful for the more obese type II diabetic.

Side effects are more common with this class of drug and include *gastrointestinal disorders, nausea, vomiting, diarrhoea, anorexia, malaise,* development of an unpleasant *metallic taste* and a risk of *lactic acidosis* (**phenformin** was withdrawn from use for this reason); metformin is not therefore recommended for elderly patients or those with hepatic or renal failure.

Oral hypoglycaemics are generally not advised to be taken during pregnancy or while breast feeding.

OTHER ANTIDIABETIC AGENTS

Acarbose (*Glucobay*) is a relatively new form of oral antidiabetic treatment. It acts as a competitive inhibitor of the α-glucosidase group of enzymes in the small intestine, which are normally responsible for the conversion of complex dietary carbohydrates like sucrose into their component monosaccharides (mainly glucose). The rise in blood glucose that follows a meal is therefore reduced. Acarbose may be taken alone with diet (50 mg tablets, three times a day before or with food) or in combination with other conventional hypoglycaemic agents. It is contraindicated for use in patients with chronic intestinal disorders or

those with hepatic/renal impairment; it is also not recommended for pregnant or nursing mothers or for children.

Side effects: these are principally gastrointestinal. The increased levels of unabsorbed carbohydrate in the bowel leads to increased production of intestinal gases, giving rise to *flatulence, abdominal distension and pain, softer stools and diarrhoea*.

Guar Gum (*Guarem*) is a non-absorbable complex carbohydrate bulking agent obtained from the seeds of the *Indian cluster bean*. When mixed with water, it forms a viscous gel that slows gastric emptying and retards intestinal carbohydrate absorption following a meal; the blood glucose level is therefore reduced. In general, consuming a relatively high proportion of dietary carbohydrate as polysaccharides has been found to improve glycaemic control in diabetics. Guar gum is available in the form of dispersable granules that are stirred into liquid and taken immediately before a main meal. It is only intended to be used as an adjunct to diet or oral hypoglycaemic therapy.

Side effects: apart from being somewhat unpalatable, guar gum preparations may cause *flatulence, abdominal distension* and a feeling of 'fullness'. It is not recommended for children.

Thiazolidinediones: These are a new class of drugs designed to facilitate insulin action. They act intracellularly beyond the insulin receptor. **Troglitazone**, representing this class, has now been approved for use in the UK and USA (marketed as *Romozin* and *Rezulin* respectively). The drug is primarily designed to break insulin resistance, and can be safely used in patients with renal failure. Food enhances its bioavailability. Treatment is initiated at 200 mg once a day, up to a maximum of 600 mg a day.

Acute Complications of Diabetic Therapy

HYPOGLYCAEMIA

A major adverse effect of the oral hypoglycaemics (particularly sulphonylureas), or injecting too much insulin, is the development of *hypoglycaemia* (blood glucose below 3 mmol/l). Patients should be warned about hypoglycaemic symptoms and advised to carry glucose tablets (*Dextrosol*) or sugar with them at all times, together with a *diabetic identity card*.

Drug interactions with the oral hypoglycaemics can also occur due to displacement of the hypoglycaemic agent from plasma protein binding by other drugs (e.g. *tolbutamide* with *aspirin* or *sulphonamides*) resulting in a sudden increase in hypoglycaemic effect. *Corticosteroids, oral contraceptives* and *thiazide diuretics* would have an opposing, i.e. *hyper*glycaemic action. Alcohol may enhance the action of insulin by exerting its own hypoglycaemic effect.

The usual autonomic (adrenergic) symptoms of acute **hypoglycaemia are:** *nervousness, sweating, tremor, palpitations* (this may be masked in patients taking *β-adrenoceptor blockers*); *intense hunger, tingling of the lips and tongue; confusion* and ultimately *loss of consciousness*; (some of these symptoms may be missed due to *autonomic neuropathy*).

☞ Since *human insulin* has a slightly more rapid onset of action and a shorter-lasting effect, some patients may experience unexpected hypoglycaemia (with less pronounced warning symptoms) on transfer from animal source to human insulin preparations.

Treatment. The immediate remedy is to take 2–4 small lumps of sugar or 3 glucose tablets with a little water at the first signs of a reaction and to lie down for 10–15 min to allow the symptoms to gradually disappear. Oral glucose should be used rather than sugar, when taking *acarbose*. If the patient is unconscious, an intramuscular injection of **glucagon** (1 mg) may be given to raise the blood glucose level, followed by oral glucose when the patient responds. If no response is obtained, then an intravenous infusion of 20–50 ml glucose (50%) should be administered.

KETOACIDOSIS AND DIABETIC COMA

Ketoacidosis develops more gradually (over a period of days) and only in type I diabetics. It can be caused by injecting too little (or no) insulin, or brought on by an acute infection, illness or sudden stress, all of which tend to increase the blood glucose level. Therefore, for insulin-dependent diabetics, it is important to continue to inject their normal, or a slightly increased insulin dose during an illness.

The usual symptoms of diabetic ketoacidosis are: *excessive thirst, frequent urination* (leading to *dehydration*); *drowsiness, abdominal pain; loss of appetite; nausea, vomiting, hyperventilation,* and a *strong smell of acetone on the breath.*

If untreated, the condition may lead to *diabetic coma* and death. It is therefore considered as a *medical emergency* and requires immediate intravenous infusion with **soluble insulin** (1 unit/ml; 0.2 units/kg body weight as a bolus, followed by 0.1 unit/kg continuous infusion) and correction fluids (*sodium chloride, potassium chloride* and *sodium bicarbonate* [when acidosis is severe]) until the blood glucose level has fallen to <10 mmol/l, blood ketones have disappeared and the patient is well enough to take food. Treatment of any underlying infection should also be ongoing. ■

Review Questions

Question 1: State from which cells of the pancreas insulin is secreted.

Question 2: State what other principal peptides are secreted by the pancreatic islet cells.

Question 3: Describe the basic molecular structure of insulin and outline its synthesis from precursor peptides.

Question 4: Describe the control of insulin release by (a) the blood glucose concentration, (b) other islet hormones, (c) gastro-intestinal hormones, (d) dietary amino acids.

Question 5: State the major action of insulin on the blood glucose level.

Question 6: State the major target organs for insulin action.

Question 7: What is the normal range of plasma glucose concentration?

Question 8: Describe the effects of insulin on glucose transport.

Question 9: State what tissues are independent of insulin for glucose transport.

Question 10: Describe the effects of insulin on:
(a) glycogen metabolism,
(b) hepatic glucose phosphorylation,
(c) liver glucose metabolism,
(d) muscle protein metabolism,
(e) fat metabolism in adipose tissue.

Question 11: State from which islet cells glucagon is secreted.

Question 12: Describe the control of glucagon release by:
(a) the blood glucose concentration,
(b) other islet hormones,
(c) gastrointestinal hormones,
(d) amino acids.

Question 13: State the major action of glucagon on the blood glucose level.

Question 14: State the major target organ for glucagon action.

Question 15: Describe the effects of glucagon action on:
(a) glycogen metabolism,
(b) fat metabolism.

Question 16: Name the condition characterized by hyposecretion of insulin.

Question 17: List the major consequences of insulin deficiency.

Question 18: Name some other hormones that may cause hyperglycaemia when secreted in excess.

Question 19: List the principal features of type I diabetes.

Question 20: List the principal features of type II diabetes.

Question 21: What is amylin? From where is it secreted, and what is its proposed role in the aetiology of type II diabetes?

Question 22: Explain the condition of gestational diabetes and how it can arise.

Question 23: Describe some common tests for monitoring urinary/blood glucose concentration and give their underlying principles of use.

Question 24: Explain the significance of glycosylated Hb as a measure of diabetic control.

Question 25: Describe the glucose tolerance test and explain the expected result for a normal or diabetic subject.

Question 26: Describe the macrovascular and microvascular complications that can arise in long-term diabetic patients.

Question 27: Describe some other chronic complications of diabetes.

Question 28: Outline the major aims of diabetic treatment.

Question 29: State the three current methods available for diabetic treatment.

Question 30: Give examples of possible treatment regimes for type I diabetes.

Question 31: Describe the use of insulin pump systems in the treatment of diabetes. What do you understand by the terms 'open loop' and 'closed loop' pump therapy?

Question 32:   Discuss the use of pancreatic islet cell transplantation as a possible approach for the treatment of diabetes.

Question 33:   Give examples of some currently available types of insulin preparation.

Question 34:   Outline possible treatment regimens for type II diabetes.

Question 35:   Give examples of some currently used oral hypoglycaemic drugs, explain their mechanism of action and give their side effects.

Question 36:   Give examples of other commonly used antidiabetic agents, and explain their mechanism of action.

Question 37:   Describe some possible drug interactions that can occur while taking oral hypoglycaemic drugs.

Question 38:   Describe the possible causes, symptoms and treatment of hypoglycaemia.

Question 39:   Describe the causes, symptoms and treatment of diabetic ketoacidosis and diabetic coma.

Question 40:   What are the causes of hyperinsulinism? List the main symptoms that may arise from this condition, and how it may be treated.

Clinical Case Studies

Patient 1

A 14 year old girl was brought to her GP's office, complaining of weight loss, dry mouth, lethargy, easy fatigability and difficulty in catching the breath; some nausea and abdominal pain was also experienced. The symptoms were noticed by the parents about 10 days before the visit. However, the patient herself had noted an increased frequency of urination (polyuria) and increased thirst (polydipsia) about 8–10 weeks prior.

A urine analysis using the *Clinitest* method and *Ketostix* reagent strips revealed positive glucose and ketones respectively. Her temperature was 39°C and a chest examination revealed some congestion. The patient was immediately admitted to hospital for management. Clinical examination revealed a dehydration, fruity odour to the breath, tachycardia (120 beats/min) and dry mouth, lips and tongue. The respiratory rate was 30/min and her blood pressure was 110/70 mmHg.

Laboratory data indicated that her plasma glucose level was 26.1 mmol/l, serum acetone was positive (at a dilution of 1:8), arterial blood pH was 7.18 with a bicarbonate level of 17 mmol/l. Other serum values determined at this time were (mmol/l): Na^+ 130, K^+ 5.8, Cl^- 92, and glycosylated haemoglobin 13.1%; blood islet cell antibodies were positive, and the HLA genotype was DR3/DR4.

Question   1:   What is the most likely diagnosis in this patient? What are the causes of her observed symptomatology ? Suggest a likely precipitating factor of her condition.

Question   2:   What would be the most appropriate treatment while in hospital, and the recommended therapy on discharge?

Answer   1:   This is a classical presentation of *diabetic ketoacidosis in insulin-dependent diabetes mellitus (IDDM, or type I diabetes)*. The common symptoms of diabetes mellitus are: *polyuria* (increased urine volume and frequency), *polydipsia* (increased thirst) and *polyphagia* (increased appetite). Polyuria is secondary to the osmotic diuresis (caused by excess filtered glucose in the urine) which then triggers increased thirst. Diabetic ketoacidosis is a serious acute complication that requires prompt attention. It is usually precipitated in insulin-dependent diabetic patients by a stressful stimulus (e.g. an infection, surgery or acute illness) or by omitting several insulin injections. The characteristic sweet smell to the breath is due to excretion of acetone (ketone body) formed by condensation of excess acetyl CoA in the liver; appearance of other ketone bodies in the blood (acetoacetate and 3-hydroxybutyrate) decreases blood pH (metabolic acidosis) which stimulates respiration (hyperventilation).

Answer 2: Following a diagnosis of diabetic ketoacidosis, intravenous fluid replacement and correction of hyperglycaemia/ketonaemia is crucial for effective hospital management; a precipitating cause such as an infection should also be sought and treated with appropriate antibiotics if necessary. The patient was started on intravenous fluid (normal saline) and soluble insulin infusion (0.2 units/kg bolus followed by 0.1 units/kg per hour) to correct for the underlying dehydration and metabolic abnormalities. In the next 14 hours, the blood glucose was stabilized at 7.8 mmol/l and the patient rehydrated. Serum electrolytes returned to normal (bicarbonate level increased to 22 mmol/l) and arterial blood pH showed normalization to 7.35. Insulin infusion was continued until next morning, when ketones were no longer present in the diluted serum. The patient was switched to subcutaneous insulin administered twice daily. She was instructed in home blood glucose monitoring methods and discharged on stable doses of insulin three days later.

Laboratory Findings

People with a DR3/DR4 HLA genotype have a high risk of developing IDDM; such individuals also commonly possess islet b-cell antibodies in their serum. Glycosylated haemoglobin (HbA$_{1C}$) levels in the blood are useful for assessing long-term glycaemic control; normal values are between 3.9–6.8% of total blood Hb.

'Normal' values for blood constituents are (mmol/l):

Na^+ 135–145; K^+ 3.5–5.0; Cl^- 98–108; HCO_3^- 22–26; glucose 3.6–6.4 (65–115 mg/dl).

The normal pH range of the blood serum is 7.42–7.38; metabolic acidosis results when the arterial blood pH is <7.38 (reflected by the low serum bicarbonate level).

Patient 2

A 49 year old male was admitted to hospital with symptoms of extreme thirst, fatigue and polyuria. Investigations were generally normal, although he had detectable glucose and protein but no ketones in his urine. A BM-Test strip test revealed a blood glucose level of 18 mmol/l. The patient was 5′8″ tall and weighed 76 kg (12 stone; 168 lb). Clinical examination revealed moderate hypertension (160/104 mmHg) and tachycardia (100 beats/min) and a soft systolic murmur in the mitral area. On enquiry, the patient mentioned that for the last 6 months he had noticed chest pain on exertion, but these episodes only lasted 5–10 min. Lately, the frequency and duration of these chest pains had increased. He also complained of nocturia (three times nightly). Blood chemistry analysis revealed a plasma glucose level of 12.1 mmol/l and a total cholesterol level of 12 mmol/l (233 mg/dl); [ideal <5.2 mmol/l (100 mg/dl)]. Glycosylated haemoglobin was 9.1% (normal <6.8%); no other abnormalities were noted.

Question 1: *What is the most likely diagnosis in this patient, and what are the causes of his symptoms? Describe the typical profile of this condition; how commonly it is encountered in the population? Is there a hereditary link?*

Question 2: *How common is hypertension or other cardiovascular problems in such patients?*

Question 3: *How is the condition treated (while in hospital, and on discharge)?*

Answer 1: This is a typical presentation of *non-insulin-dependent diabetes mellitus (NIDDM, or type II diabetes)*, where hyperglycaemia is discovered on blood chemistry analysis. It is the more common form of diabetes, but is normally slower to develop, usually in older (>40 years) more obese individuals. As in type I diabetes, increased urination (polyuria), is due to glucose-induced osmotic diuresis, which causes an increase in plasma osmolarity and a consequent stimulation of the thirst centre in the brain (polydipsia); ketosis, however, is typically absent. A strong genetic link exists in the development of NIDDM.

Answer 2: Many patients will have macrovascular disease (coronary artery disease, cerebrovascular disease) and a high blood cholesterol level (*hypercholesterolaemia*) at the time of presentation. Hypertension is about twice as common in persons with diabetes as in those without the condition, essential hypertension accounting for the majority of the cases encountered. 30–75% of chronic diabetic complications can be attributed to hypertension.

Answer 3: On diagnosis of NIDDM, diet, exercise and weight reduction can be very effective in the treatment of mild cases, and may assist in lowering the blood pressure in associated hypertension. Use of *oral hypoglycaemic drugs* may also help to produce adequate glycaemic control in the vast majority of NIDDM cases; however, insulin will invariably be required to control the diabetes more effectively, particularly if oral hypoglycaemics have been used for five or more years. While in the hospital, the patient was placed on a 1600 calorie diet and given subcutaneous insulin to control his blood glucose; subsequently, he was switched to oral hypoglycaemic medication (*glipizide 5 mg, twice daily*). His blood glucose was normalized, with post-prandial blood glucose rarely exceeding 7.8 mmol/l. Meanwhile, further clinical examination revealed significant and diffuse coronary artery disease.

Patient 3

A 35 year old female who was 29 weeks pregnant attended her local GP's office for a routine checkup. Her GP noted glycosuria and a larger than normal foetus for gestational date, and referred her urgently to the antenatal clinic. The patient weighed 10.5 stone (147 lb; 66.8 kg) prior to pregnancy, and had no previous history of diabetes, but her two previous babies weighed 9 lb and 10 lb at birth. At the clinic, an *oral glucose tolerance test (OGTT)* was given, with the following results:

Fasting (venous) plasma glucose	10.7 mmol/l
30 min post test	21.5 mmol/l
120 min post test	19.2 mmol/l

Question 1: *What is the oral glucose tolerance test and what does it involve? How useful is it in the diagnosis of diabetes?*

Question 2: *What is the most likely diagnosis in this patient, and how should her condition be managed? What are the risk factors associated with its development?*

Question 3: *What are the implications of leaving the condition untreated or inadequately managed?*

Question 4: *How likely is it that her condition will resolve after delivery?*

Answer 1: The *oral glucose tolerance test (OGTT)* is a useful and reliable diagnostic test for diabetes, which measures the ability of an overnight-fasted subject to handle an ingested glucose load (75 g) over a 2–3 hour period. Plasma glucose levels are measured at zero time and then every half hour for 2–3 hours after the glucose challenge. In non-diabetics, the plasma glucose should not exceed 8.5 mmol/l during the test, and should return to normal fasting levels (ca. 4–6 mmol/l; <110 mg/dl) after 2 hours. In a diabetic patient, a high fasting plasma glucose (>7.8 mmol/l) and a higher, more prolonged peak glucose level (>11.1 mmol/l) is observed.

Answer 2: This patient has developed *gestational diabetes* during pregnancy, diagnosed from the abnormally high fasting and two hour plasma glucose concentrations seen during the *OGTT*. Women that are obese (weight >120% of normal for height), with a family history of diabetes, or showing previous symptoms of glucose intolerance are particularly at risk of developing the condition; so also are women with a poor obstetric history i.e. previous babies >9 lb at birth, or present foetus larger than normal for gestational age (macrosomia), unexplained foetal deaths or infants with congenital abnormalities. Such women also have a high probability of developing type II diabetes (NIDDM) at a future date.

Answer 3: Even mild diabetes developing during pregnancy can significantly increase the risk of major foetal abnormalities (particularly in the cardiovascular and central nervous systems) or foetal death. Leaving gestational diabetes untreated or poor management can also increase the maternal risk of infection, hyperglycaemia, diabetic ketoacidosis, retinopathy, nephropathy or neuropathy. The patient was prescribed biphasic isophane insulin (*Human Mixtard 30 pen*), 18 units daily (12 units with breakfast, and six units with dinner) adjusted throughout the pregnancy according to self-monitored blood glucose levels. The goal was to achieve postprandial blood glucose measurements between 4–10 mmol/l. She was also placed on a reduced calorie diet (1500–1800 daily) and advised to avoid sugary and fatty foods in favour of more complex carbohydrates. Her random blood glucose measurement at 32 weeks was 7.8 mmol/l.

Answer 4: The likelihood of gestational diabetes resolving after delivery is very good (>90%); however, the risk of recurrence during a subsequent pregnancy or development of NIDDM at a future date remains high (ca. 50% risk). Careful blood glucose monitoring after delivery is therefore advisable.

UK/USA Drugs — Trade names		
	UK	**USA**
Oral hypoglycaemic drugs		
Acetohexamide		Dymelor
Chlorpropamide	Diabinese	Diabenese
Glibenclamide	Daonil	
Gliclazide	Diamicron	
Glipizide	Glibenese	Glucotrol
Glyburide		DiaBeta/Glynase
		Micronase
Metformin	Glucophage	Glucophage
Tolazamide		Tolinase
Tolbutamide	Rastinon	Orinase
Antidiabetic agents		
Acarbose	Glucobay	Precose
Guar gum	Guarem	
Troglitazone	Romozin	Rezulin

Insulin preparations — USA trade names	
Short-acting insulins	*Intermediate-acting insulins*
Humulin R	Humulin L,N
Iletin I	Iletin I, Lente
Novolin R	Insulatard
Regular insulin	Lente insulin
Semilente insulin	Novolin L,N
Velosulin	
Humalog (Insulin Lys-Pro)	
Long-acting insulins	*Premixed*
Humulin U	Humulin 50/50, 70/30
Ultralente insulin	Mixtard 70/30
	Novolin 70/40

References

Books

- **Cawson RA, McCracken AW, Marcus PB, Zaatari GS.** (1989). Diseases of the endocrine system. In *Pathology. The mechanisms of disease*, 2nd ed. CV. Mosby Co, 434–460
- **Chandrasoma P, Taylor CR.** (1991). The endocrine pancreas. In *Concise Pathology*, 1st ed, Prentice-Hall, USA, pp. 677–687
- **Davis SN, Granner DK.** (1996). Insulin, oral hypoglycemic agents and the pharmacology of the endocrine pancreas. In *Goodman & Gilman's The Pharmacological Basis of Therapeutics*, edited by JG Hardman, LE Limbird, A Goodman, Gilman *et al.*, 9th ed. McGraw-Hill, USA, pp. 1487–1517
- **Foster DW, McGarry JD.** (1988). Glucose, lipid and protein metabolism. In *Textbook of Endocrine Physiology*, edited by JE Griffin, SR Ojeda. Oxford University Press, New York, pp. 302–326
- **Ganong WF.** (1995). Endocrine functions of the pancreas & the regulation of carbohydrate metabolism. In *Review of Medical Physiology*, 17th ed. Appleton & Lange, Connecticut, pp. 306–326
- **Genuth SM.** (1993). Hormones of the pancreatic islets. In *Physiology*, edited by RM Berne, MN Levy, 3rd ed. Mosby-Year Book Inc, USA, pp. 851–875
- **Goodman HM.** (1988). Islets of Langerhans. In *Basic Medical Endocrinology*. Raven Press, New York, pp. 115–141
- **Greene RJ, Harris ND, Goodyer LI.** (1993). Major pathological processes in disease. In *Pathology and Therapeutics of Pharmacists*. Chapman & Hall, London, pp. 29–31
- **Guyton AC, Hall JE.** (1996). Insulin, glucagon and diabetes mellitus. In *Textbook of Medical Physiology*, 9th ed. WB Saunders Company, USA, pp. 971–983
- **Hassan T.** (1985). Diabetes mellitus. In *A Guide to Medical Endocrinology*. Macmillan Publishers Ltd, pp. 87–123
- **Hillson RM.** (1994). The drug therapy of endocrine and metabolic disorders. In *Oxford Texbook of Clinical Pharmacology and Drug Therapy*, edited by DG Grahame-Smith, JK Aronson, 2nd ed. Oxford University Press, pp. 365–398
- **Junqueira LC, Carneiro J, Long JA.** (1986). Adrenals & other endocrine glands. In *Basic Histology*, 5th ed. Lange Medical Publications, Connecticut, pp. 446–467
- **Karam JH, Forsham PH.** (1994). Pancreatic hormones & Diabetes Mellitus. In *Basic & Clinical Endocrinology*, edited by FS Greenspan, JD Baxter, 4th ed. Appleton & Lange, Connecticut, pp. 571–634
- **Koda-Kimble MA.** (1975). Diabetes mellitus. In *Applied Therapeutics for Clinical Pharmacists*, edited by MA Koda-Kimble, BS Katcher, LY Young, 2nd ed. Applied Therapeutics Inc, San Francisco, pp. 449–493
- **Kumar PJ, Clark ML.** (1990). Diabetes mellitus and other disorders of metabolism. In *Clinical Medicine*, 2nd ed. Bailliere Tindall, pp. 832–872

- **Laurence DR, Bennett PN.** (1992). Endocrinology II: diabetes mellitus, insulin, oral antidiabetic agents. In *Clinical Pharmacology*. Churchill Livingstone, pp. 565–580
- **Longhurst PA.** (1987). Pancreatic hormones. In *Clinical Endocrine Physiology*. WB Saunders Co, Philadelphia, pp. 265–295
- **Lorenzi M.** (1992). Diabetes mellitus. In *Handbook of Clinical Endocrinology*, edited by PA Fitzgerald, 2nd ed. Prentice-Hall, USA, pp. 463–560
- **Mulvihill SJ, Debas HT.** (1994). Regulatory peptides of the gut. In *Basic & Clinical Endocrinology*, edited by FS Greenspan, JD Baxter, 4th ed. Appleton & Lange, Connecticut, pp. 551–570
- **Rang HP, Dale MM, Ritter JM.** (1995). The endocrine pancreas and the control of blood glucose. In *Pharmacology*, 3rd ed. Churchill Livingstone, pp. 403–416
- **Rees PJ, Williams DG.** (1995). Disorders of metabolism. In *Principles of Clinical Medicine*. Edward Arnold, pp. 475–516
- **Watkins PJ.** (1993). *ABC of Diabetes*, 3rd ed. BMJ Publishing Group, London
- **Whitby LG, Percy-Robb IW, Smith AF.** (1984). Disorders of carbohydrate metabolism. In *Lecture Notes on Clinical Chemistry*, 3rd ed. Blackwell Scientific Publications, Oxford, pp. 213–241

Journal Articles

- **Al-Habori M.** (1993). Mechanism of insulin action, role of ions and the cytoskeleton. *Int J Biochem*, 25, 1087–1099
- **Amoroso S, Schmid-Antomarchi H** *et al.* (1990). Glucose, sulfonylureas and neurotransmitter release: role of ATP-sensitive K$^+$ channels. *Science*, 247, 852–854
- **Backer JM, Myers MG Jr, Shoelson SE** *et al.* (1992). Phosphatidylinositol 3'-kinase is activated by association with IRS-1 during insulin stimulation. *EMBO J*, 11, 3469–3479
- **Becker AB, Roth RA.** (1990). Insulin receptor structure and function in normal and pathological conditions. *Annu Rev Med*, 41, 99–115
- **Brange J, Owens DR** *et al.* (1990). Monomeric insulins and their experimental and clinical implications. *Diabetes Care*, 13, 923–954
- **Campbell I.** (1994). Diabetes and the role of oral hypoglycaemic drugs. *Prescriber*, 5(5), 63–68
- **Cheatham B, Kahn CR.** (1995). Insulin action and the insulin signaling network. *Endocrine Rev*, 16, 117–142
- **Clauser E, Leconte I, Auzan I.** (1992). Molecular basis of insulin resistance. *Hormone Res*, 38, 5–12
- **Cohick WS, Clemmons DR.** (1993). The insulin-like growth factors. *Annu Rev Physiol*, 55, 131–153
- **Daneman D.** (1994). Glycated hemoglobin in the assessment of diabetes control. *The Endocrinologist*, 4, 33–43

- **DelValle J, Yamada T.** (1990). The gut as an endocrine organ. *Annu Rev Med*, 41, 447–455
- **Dent P, Lavoinne A** *et al.* (1990). The molecular mechanism by which insulin stimulates glycogen synthesis in mammalian skeletal muscle. *Nature*, 348, 302–308
- **Ellison EC, Johnson JA.** (1994). Gastrointestinal peptides: basic physiology and clinical significance. *Prob Gen Surg*, 11, 1–20
- **Kimbal SR, Vary TC, Jefferson LS.** (1994). Regulation of protein synthesis by insulin. *Annu Rev Physiol*, 56, 321–348
- **Lacy PE.** (1995). Treating diabetes with transplanted cells. *Scientific American*, July 1995, 40–46
- **Lawrence JC Jr.** (1992). Signal transduction and protein phosphorylation in the regulation of cellular metabolism by insulin. *Annu Rev Physiol*, 54, 177–193
- **Lorenzo A, Razzaboni B** *et al.* (1994). Pancreatic islet cell toxicity of amylin associated with type-2 diabetes mellitus. *Nature*, 368, 756–760
- **MacRury S.** (1992). The control of noninsulin-dependent diabetes. *Prescriber*, 3(10), 59–63
- **Myers MG Jr, White MF.** (1996). Insulin signal transduction and the IRS proteins. *Ann Rev Pharmacol Toxicol*, 36, 615–658
- **Perros P, Frier B.** (1993). Making effective use of insulins in diabetes. *Prescriber*, 4(20), 27–32
- **Pessin JE, Bell GI.** (1992). Mammalian facilitative glucose transporter family: structure and molecular regulation. *Annu Rev Physiol*, 54, 911–930
- **Rink TJ, Beaumont K** *et al.* (1993). Structure and biology of amylin. *Trends in Pharmacol Sci*, 14, 113–118
- **Sanchez MV, Valle M** *et al.* (1995). Plasma pancreastatin-like immunoreactivity correlates with plasma norepinephrine levels in essential hypertension. *Neuropeptides*, 29, 97–101
- **Scheen AJ.** (1997). Drug treatment of non-insulin-dependent diabetes mellitus in the 1990s: Achievements and future developments. *Drugs*, 54, 355–368
- **Strålfors P.** (1997). Insulin second messengers. *BioEssays*, 19, 327–335
- **Tamada JA, Bohannon NJV, Potts RO.** (1995). Measurement of glucose in diabetic subjects using noninvasive transdermal extraction. *Nature Med*, 1, 1198–1201
- **Thorsby E, Undlien D.** (1996). The HLA associated predisposition to type 1 diabetes and other autoimmune diseases. *J Pediat Endocrinol Metab*, 9, 75–88
- **Wales J.** (1994). Acarbose — a new type of oral antidiabetic agent. *Prescriber*, 5(3), 19–24
- **White MF, Kahn CR.** (1994). The insulin signaling system. *J Biol Chem*, 269, 1–4
- **Zick Y.** (1989). The insulin receptor: structure and function. *Crit Rev Biochem Molec Biol*, 24, 217–269
- **Zimmerman BR.** (1994). Glycaemia control in diabetes mellitus: towards the normal profile? *Drugs*, 47, 611–621

6 | The Gonads and Reproduction

The Gonads (i.e. *ovaries* in the female, and the *testes* in the male) serve two main functions:

1. to produce *germ* cells (ova or sperm) – *gametogenesis*
2. to produce certain *steroid sex hormones* necessary for normal development and function of the reproductive organs and differentiation of secondary sex characteristics. They also have an important role during pregnancy, parturition (childbirth) and lactation.

There are three types of sex hormone secreted:

1. **Androgens** – male sex hormones – e.g. **Testosterone**
2. **Oestrogens** – female sex hormones – e.g. **17β-Oestradiol**
3. **Progestogens** – female sex hormones – e.g. **Progesterone**

Androgens and *oestrogens* exert masculinizing or feminizing effects in the body respectively, whereas *progestogens* mainly affect the uterus in preparation for and during pregnancy (Figure 6.1).

While *the testes* continuously produce spermatozoa and **testosterone** from puberty (ca. 13 years) to old age, in the adult female, usually only one ovum is produced approximately every 28 days, and **oestrogen/progesterone** secretion occurs cyclically (*the menstrual cycle*) until the *menopause*, when the ovarian cycle ceases.

The functioning of the gonads and sexual function is primarily controlled by the hypothalamus and anterior pituitary, under the influence of higher brain centres (the cortex).

Puberty is most probably initiated by a maturation and 'release from inhibition' of the hypothalamic **gonadotrophin releasing hormone (GnRH)** neurones of the arcuate nucleus, leading to gradual establishment of *pulsatile* GnRH release (frequency about 60–90 mins) and a consequent increase in pulsatile gonadotrophin secretion from the pituitary. Premature activation of this hypothalamic-pituitary system (e.g. caused by a brain tumour or hydrocephalus) may lead to *precocious puberty* in children.

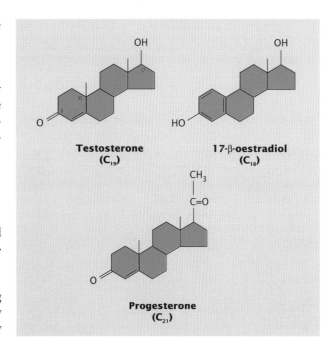

Figure 6.1. Structures of the principal steroid sex hormones secreted by the testes in males (testosterone) or by the ovaries in females (17β-oestradiol and progesterone). All bear the same characteristic 4-ringed nucleus (derived from cholesterol). Note that testosterone and progesterone differ only in the type of grouping attached at position C_{17}, whereas oestradiol lacks the methyl group at position C_{10}.

The Male Reproductive System
Structure and Histology

Like the female ovary, the testes have both an endocrine and exocrine function. Each testis (about 20 g) situated in the *scrotum*, is largely composed of numerous coiled *seminiferous tubules* surrounded by a fibrous capsule; the inner walls of these tubules contain a large number of spermatogenic cells (*spermatogonia, spermatocytes* and *spermatids*) that undergo various stages of division and development to produce *spermatozoa* (an *exocrine-holocrine* secretion). The tubular epithelium also contains larger *Sertoli cells* (extending from the basal membrane to the tubular lumen) that are involved in supporting and nourishing the sperm cells during their process of maturation. *Tight junctions* present between adjacent Sertoli cells form a 'blood-testes barrier' (separating *basal* and *adluminal* compartments of the tubule) that creates a unique environment for more advanced germ cells, and may protect them from possible noxious substances in the general circulation. Fully-formed spermatozoa (about $100–200 \times 10^6$/day) are released from the apex of the Sertoli cells into the lumen of the seminiferous tubules.

Lying in between the seminiferous tubules, together with blood vessels, lymphatics and nerves, are groups of interstitial *Leydig cells* which synthesize and secrete **testosterone** into the circulation. Sertoli cells are also capable of converting androgens to oestrogens, which may exert a localized paracrine function on Leydig cells to limit testosterone production. Most (about 70%) of the oestrogen present in the circulation of adult men is, however, non-testicular – derived from circulating testosterone and androstenedione through *aromatase* enzyme activity in peripheral tissues (mainly adipose tissue and liver); the rate of extraglandular oestrogen production tends to increase with age.

☞ Brain aromatization of testosterone (released by the foetal testis) to 17β-oestradiol within the foetal hypothalamus, is thought to be responsible for the early differentiation of the 'male-type' hypothalamic/pituitary negative feedback axis. The aromatase enzyme system is also found in other brain areas, suggesting a more general role for locally-formed oestrogens in prenatal brain development.

Control of Spermatogenesis and Hormone Release

Testicular function is regulated primarily by the release of anterior pituitary gonadotrophins, LH and FSH, which in turn, is driven by hypothalamic GnRH. The initiation and maintenance of spermatogenesis by the seminiferous tubules requires the action of both LH and FSH. FSH action on the Sertoli cells is particularly important for the initiation of spermatogenesis. Afterwards, LH assumes more importance by stimulating the Leydig cells to produce testosterone, which diffuses to adjacent Sertoli cells and has a key role in the maintenance of spermatogenesis. Testosterone is important for the final development of spermatids into spermatozoa. FSH together with testosterone, also stimulate the Sertoli cells to produce

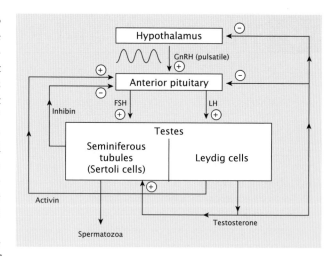

Figure 6.2. Control of testosterone secretion by the testes. Pulsatile release of gonadotrophin releasing hormone (GnRH) by the hypothalamus, stimulates the secretion of the gonadotrophins luteinizing hormone (LH) and follicle stimulating hormone (FSH) from the anterior pituitary. LH stimulates the testicular Leydig cells to produce testosterone, which in turn diffuses to adjacent Sertoli cells to affect spermatogenesis and also exerts negative feedback effects on the hypothalamus and pituitary. FSH release is regulated by the production of peptide factors inhibin and activin by the tubular Sertoli cells or Leydig cells respectively, which have a direct negative or positive feedback action on the pituitary.

androgen binding protein (ABP) which sequesters testosterone in the tubular lumen fluid and thus helps to maintain a high intratubular concentration of the hormone, necessary for normal spermatogenesis. The actions of FSH are mediated via specific FSH receptors (linked to cAMP production) located primarily, if not exclusively, on the Sertoli cells. LH and FSH in addition, exert important trophic (growth-promoting) effects on the Leydig cells and Sertoli cells respectively.

CONTROL OF RELEASE

The production of **testosterone** is controlled principally by LH acting on the Leydig cells; this effect is mediated by surface LH receptors coupled to intracellular cAMP production. Testosterone inhibits LH release by direct and indirect negative feedback loops acting on the anterior pituitary and hypothalamus respectively (Figure 6.2). It does not, however, reduce FSH release at normal levels. A peptide hormone **inhibin**, secreted by the Sertoli cells under the influence of FSH (see Chapter 2) is believed to exert this effect by a direct negative feedback action on the pituitary.

☞ **Inhibin** is a dimeric 32-kDa glycoprotein consisting of two dissimilar subunits, α and β; (two forms of the β chain, A and B are produced). Interestingly, a second structurally related gonadal peptide, **activin**, formed from two inhibin β chains, has the *opposite* effects to inhibin on pituitary FSH release and on gonadal steroidogenesis. In males, activin is secreted predominantly by the testicular Leydig cells. Inhibin and activin may produce important local (*paracrine*) effects on neighbouring Leydig and Sertoli cells; the two peptides may also have important regulatory functions outside the reproductive system e.g. in controlling early cellular differentiation and development. An inhibin-like peptide is known to be secreted by the adrenal glands, and may be important in adrenocortical cell proliferation and/or differentiation. A possible use of inhibin as a male contraceptive agent has been suggested.

A monomeric glycoprotein **follistatin**, also found in ovarian follicular fluid, has a similar (though less potent) inhibitory effect to inhibin on pituitary FSH release, but is structurally unrelated to the inhibin or activin molecules. Follistatin binds circulating activin with high affinity and can therefore neutralise and limit its biological effects in many tissues; the significance of follistatin in human reproduction is, however, unclear.

Androgens: Testosterone

The main steroid hormone secreted by the testes is **testosterone** (synthesized largely from low density lipoprotein [LDL]-cholesterol, converted to pregnenolone; c.f. adrenal steroids: Chapter 3). Small amounts of testosterone are also secreted by the adrenal cortex (in both males and females) and also by the ovaries in females. About 98% of plasma testosterone is protein bound: 65% to a *sex hormone binding globulin (SHBG)* (synthesized by the liver) and the remainder to albumin and other proteins. The plasma half-life of unbound (biologically-active) testosterone is only about 10–20 min, most being rapidly metabolized by the liver to inactive *17-ketosteroids* (mainly *androsterone* and *etiocholanolone*) and also to polar metabolites (-diols, -triols and conjugates [glucuronides and sulphates]) and excreted in the urine. Since albumin-bound testosterone is readily dissociable, the amount of 'bioavailable' testosterone is considered as being the sum of the unbound and albumin-bound hormone.

Testosterone stimulates the growth and development of the entire male genital tract; it also has potent *protein anabolic* properties (increase in synthesis of protein, leading to an increase in muscle mass and nitrogen retention).

The principal effects of testosterone may be summarized as follows:

1. *In the foetus*, testosterone, secreted by the embryonic testes during a critical foetal period (8–12 weeks), is responsible for differentiation of the male internal and external genitalia and for promoting the descent of the testes into the scrotum (*müllerian inhibiting substance* secreted by the foetal testes prevents development of female genital ducts in the male foetus; see below).

2. *During puberty*, it is responsible for the growth of the male sex organs, and contributes to the pubertal 'growth spurt' (accelerated growth phase) and eventual fusion of the bone ends (*epiphyses*) of the long bones (cessation of growth at adult height); it also causes deepening of the voice (due to enlargement of the vocal cords), growth of facial, pubic, axillary (armpit) and body hair, as well as an increase in muscularity and strength. An increase in secretory activity of the sebaceous glands of the face may lead to acne.

3. *In the adult*, it maintains masculinity as well as libido (sexual drive) and sexual potency; its role in the maintenance of the erectile response is controversial. Along with FSH, it is required to regulate spermatogenesis in the testes, and exerts an important feedback effect on the hypothalamus and pituitary (Figure 6.2). Testosterone is also responsible for recession of the scalp and baldness in genetically disposed individuals. A slight decline in bioavailable testosterone level occurs with age in healthy men (about 1% per year, between 40 and 70 years), but there is no abrupt decrease analogous to the female menopause.

MECHANISM OF ACTION

As with other steroid hormones (see Chapter 3), the actions of testosterone are mediated directly via an intracellular high affinity *androgen receptor protein (AR)* that ultimately binds to specific *androgen-responsive elements (AREs)* on the nuclear DNA; this affects transcription (either positively or negatively) of specific genes and therefore synthesis of specific proteins within the cell cytoplasm. Conversion of testosterone to the more potent 5α-**dihydrotestosterone (DHT)** however, occurs in some target tissues (particularly skin, prostate gland and seminal vesicles), catalysed by the nuclear enzyme *5-α-reductase*. DHT interacts with the same intracellular receptor as testosterone, but has a two-fold higher binding affinity, and a slower rate of dissociation; it exerts significant androgenic activity at these sites. Thus, in addition to its direct effects, testosterone serves as a *prohormone* for intracellular DHT production within specific androgen target tissues.

Differentiation of the male external genitalia and prostate gland in the foetus requires the action of DHT rather than testosterone, whereas the latter is important for mediating the development of the wolffian ducts into the male internal genitalia. DHT is also the active hormone responsible for prostate and penile growth at puberty as well as development of facial hair, acne and possible scalp recession in later life.

In women, **androstendione** is the major precursor of DHT production in the skin. Unlike testosterone, DHT is a non-aromatizable androgen; i.e. it is not a substrate for aromatase, therefore cannot be converted peripherally to oestrogens.

☞ In the male embryo during development, immature Sertoli cells secrete an inhibin-like peptide, **müllerian inhibiting substance (MIS)**, responsible for causing regression of the müllerian duct system, that would otherwise develop into fallopian tubes and a uterus. MIS is a glycoprotein dimer that belongs to the *transforming growth factor-beta (TGF-β)* superfamily of peptides (including *activin*, and *inhibin*), involved in regulating cell growth and differentiation; it requires enzymatic cleavage by a protease to become biologically active. MIS is also present in the testes postnatally for several years (up to and including early puberty), before declining to low levels. In females, it can be found in the ovaries, but not until the onset of puberty; thereafter it continues to be synthesized by the ovarian granulosa cells throughout reproductive life and may therefore be important in controlling oocyte maturation. The measurement of serum MIS levels can be useful in diagnosing patients showing a variety of congenital intersex and gonadal abnormalities. In addition, *recombinant human MIS (rhMIS)* has been shown to cause regression of certain gynaecological tumours *in vitro*, and may therefore have a clinical use in the future, as a novel anticancer treatment.

Clinical Disorders

Hyposecretion or hypofunction of testosterone in the male (*hypogonadism*) may result from several types of abnormality:

1. Absence of functional testes at birth (e.g. due to *chromosomal abnormalities: primary hypogonadism*).
2. Underdevelopment of testes due to inadequate secretion of pituitary gonadotrophins (*hypopituitarism: secondary hypogonadism*).
3. Non-descent of foetal testes from abdomen into scrotum (*cryptorchidism*).
4. Loss of testes either prior to or following puberty (*castration* or *testicular destruction* by disease).

Loss of testicular function prior to puberty would lead to failure of normal development of the sexual organs and secondary sexual characteristics. In adults, a decrease in libido, some regression of masculine characteristics, and sterility would result.

Treatment of hypogonadism will require androgen replacement therapy, depending on the underlying cause and age of onset. Cryptorchidism may be treated (before puberty) by intramuscular administration of gonadotrophin (*Pregnyl*; see below) or by surgery.

Congenital absence of enzymes involved in testosterone action (e.g. *5-α-reductase deficiency: male pseudohermaphroditism*), or molecular defects at the testosterone receptor (or post-receptor) level (*androgen resistance*) may also cause serious abnormalities in sexual development. In the former case, genotypic males show female appearance with ambiguous external genitalia throughout childhood, but undergo progressive virilization at puberty, due to increased levels of testosterone. Development of facial hair and acne (dependent on DHT production) are notably absent. The condition is characterized by an abnormally high plasma testosterone:DHT ratio and may require therapy with high doses of testosterone to promote penile growth.

Hypersecretion of testosterone, although extremely rare, can result from the development of Leydig cell tumours in young children, leading to a *pseudo-precocious* puberty and a premature closure of the bony epiphyses (with resultant short stature). Treatment would involve the surgical removal of the testicular tumour followed by replacement therapy if necessary.

Some Clinical Uses of Androgens

Testosterone itself cannot be given orally, because of rapid metabolism by the liver. However depot (slow release) preparations of **testosterone esters** e.g. **testosterone enanthate** (*Primoteston Depot*) or **propionate** (*Virormone*) may be given by deep intramuscular injection every 2–3 weeks, or the patient can be treated orally using capsules containing an oily solution of **testosterone undecanoate** (*Restandol*). More longer-acting depot preparations comprising of a mixture of testosterone esters (*propionate, phenylpropionate* and *isocaproate [Sustanon 100/250]*) are also available. The only other orally-active androgenic steroid currently marketed in the UK is **Mesterolone** (*Pro-Viron*). Fluoxymesterone, and methyltestosterone are used in the USA. Transdermal delivery systems are also now available (*Andropatch*) consisting of testosterone-loaded films, applied each day to scrotal or non-scrotal skin (e.g. back, abdomen, thighs, or upper arms) in the form of a patch; local skin irritation and discomfort may however occur as side effects.

Androgens may be used for:

1. *Replacement therapy* in castrated adult males, and for treatment of hypogonadism due to testicular or pituitary insufficiency; in the latter case, androgen therapy would begin at puberty (often in combination with ongoing growth hormone therapy), to promote the growth spurt and normal development of sexual characteristics. Treatment of boys must be carefully monitored to avoid premature closure of the epiphyses. Androgens are not generally used as a treatment for decreased libido and impotence (unless associated with established hypogonadism).

2. *As protein anabolic agents* to increase muscle mass after a chronic debilitating or wasting disease (e.g. severe ulcerative colitis), major surgery or in terminal conditions. Synthetic analogues (so called *anabolic steroids*) designed to have less androgenic and more anabolic effects are preferred (e.g. **nandrolone** (*Deca-Durabolin*) or **stanozolol** (*Stromba*)). The anabolic action also involves a remineralization of bone, which may become partly demineralized in some androgen-deficient men with age (osteoporosis).

Although controversial, the use of anabolic steroids for the treatment of *aplastic anaemia* is still considered useful (*erythropoietic* effect); the use of these agents by body builders or athletes, to increase aggressiveness, muscle strength, and athletic performance however, is considered unjustified and is illegal. High doses of anabolic and androgenic steroids used for this purpose can have serious adverse effects on the liver and the cardiovascular system (see below).

☞ **Erythropoietin (EPO)** is a glycoprotein hormone secreted mainly by glomerular epithelial cells of the kidney (and also by the liver), that stimulates the formation of red blood cells from precursor stem cells of the bone marrow. Its synthesis is stimulated by tissue hypoxia (resulting from anaemia, high altitude or inadequate haemoglobin oxygenation) and also by androgenic steroids (oestrogens *inhibit* erythropoiesis). **Recombinant human erythropoietin (rHuEPO)** (*Eprex; Recormon*: given by intravenous or subcutaneous injection) is now available for treatment of secondary anaemia due to chronic renal failure (in dialysis patients).

3. *Oestrogen-dependent tumour therapy*: certain advanced breast carcinomas or cervical cancers in women may undergo regression when exposed to androgens. Masculinizing side effects are however inevitable, including growth of facial hair, interruption of the menstrual cycle, deepening of the voice and development of acne.

Other general side effects associated with androgen therapy include: possible *liver damage, hepatic tumours* and *cholestatic jaundice, weight gain* with oedema due to Na^+/H_2O retention (especially in patients with heart or kidney disease), *priapism* (persistent abnormal erection) and a *decrease in male fertility* (due to a negative feedback effect on GnRH and gonadotrophin release). Suppression of spermatogenesis and decrease of testicular size during treatment with these compounds is normally reversible upon cessation of therapy.

The *anti-androgenic* compounds **cyproterone acetate** (*Androcur; Cyprostat*), **flutamide** (*Drogenil*) and **bicalutamide** (*Casodex*) are competitive antagonists of testosterone at the androgen receptor sites, and may be used to suppress excessive sexual drive in certain men (sex offenders; *Androcur*), or in combination with an oestrogen (*Dianette*) in the treatment of severe acne/hirsutism in women. Certain advanced androgen-dependent prostatic cancers (see below) may also respond favourably to anti-androgen therapy (*Casodex*).

Side effects associated with their use in men include: possible *breast growth (gynaecomastia), reversible infertility* (due to inhibition of spermatogenesis), *tiredness, depression*, and development of *osteoporosis*. Cyproterone is not currently approved for use in the USA.

Finasteride (*Proscar*) is a selective inhibitor of the *5-α-reductase* enzyme responsible for the peripheral conversion of testosterone into DHT. Since DHT is involved in normal prostatic growth and function, the inhibitor is used in the treatment of *benign prostatic hyperplasia (BPH)* to induce a shrinkage of the enlarged prostate gland and to improve urinary flow rate; several months of treatment may however, be required before any benefit is observed. BPH is a quite common, nonmalignant condition that can affect about 80% of men over 60 years of age. *Impotence* and a *decreased libido* may also occur as side effects.

The selective α_1-adrenoreceptor blockers **alfuzosin** (*Xatral SR*), **doxazosin** (*Cardura*), **indoramin** (*Doralese*) and **tamsulosin** (*Flowmaz MR*) (selective for the α_{1A} receptor subtype, predominant in the prostate) are also used in the treatment of BPH, to increase urinary flow rate and reduce obstructive symptoms.

The Female Reproductive System
Structure and Histology

The two ovaries lie either side of the uterus, close to the open ends of the oviducts (fallopian tubes) in the pelvis. Each ovary (ca. 15 g) is enveloped in a protective capsule of connective tissue and consists of a *cortex* containing many thousands of *primordial follicles* (about 200,000 at puberty) embedded in supportive tissue (the *stroma*). Each primordial follicle comprises an *ovum (oocyte)* surrounded by a single layer of epithelial *granulosa cells*. Throughout the reproductive life of the female, only about 450 of these follicles may develop to maturity and expel an oocyte, the rest undergo spontaneous degeneration (*atresia*). At the menopause (when menstruation ceases) only a few primordial follicles are present in the ovaries.

The Ovarian Cycle and Hormone Release

With each phase of the menstrual cycle, ovarian follicles go through three stages of development, the final *mature* follicle being termed a *Graafian follicle*. At the beginning (day 1) of each menstrual cycle (*follicular phase*), a group of about 10–20 primordial follicles, stimulated by the increasing FSH concentration, enlarge to form *secondary follicles* (recruitment) although after about day 6, only one usually becomes dominant and matures fully. The remaining follicles regress i.e. become *atretic*. In mid-cycle (day 14), the Graafian follicle migrates to the edge of the ovary and ruptures, liberating the oocyte into the abdominal cavity (*ovulation*) from where it enters one of the fallopian tubes. If the ovum is subsequently fertilized during its 3–4 day passage down a fallopian tube, cellular division begins (*blastocyst* stage) before implantation in the uterus, and further cell development (*trophoblast stage*). Trophoblast cells, together with adjacent blastocyst and endometrial cells, divide rapidly to form the placenta. After about 72 hours, if not fertilized, the ovum dies and is ultimately expelled through the vagina.

The process of follicular maturation may be summarized as follows:

1. *Primary (primordial) follicle* (ca. 25 mm diameter). An immature oocyte surrounded by a single follicular epithelial cell layer.
2. *Secondary follicle* (ca. 500 mm diameter). The oocyte increases in diameter and under the influence of FSH, the follicular cells multiply to form a layer of *granulosa cells*. A fluid-filled cavity (the *antrum*) appears, containing a cocktail of nutritive substances. Like the male Sertoli cells, the granulosa cells develop gap junctions between them, thus forming a protective barrier around the oocyte.
3. *Graafian follicle* (ca. 20 mm diameter). The antrum enlarges further and an outer layer of *thecal* cells develops from the ovarian stroma, which on stimulation by LH, are responsible for initiating production of **oestrogens**; these are essential for preparing the female reproductive tract for conception. The thecal cells make androgens (mainly **androstenedione**) which are ultimately converted (via *aromatase* enzyme activity) to oestrogens by the granulosa cells (stimulated by FSH and LH). Both of these effects involve a rise in intracellular cAMP.

☞ FSH (together with oestrogens) increases the number of LH and FSH receptors on granulosa cells, thereby enhancing their LH/FSH sensitivity.

After ovulation (*luteal phase*), the granulosa and theca cells of the collapsed, haemorrhaged follicle proliferate to form a yellowish *corpus luteum* (ca. 1.5 cm diameter) which, in the non-pregnant woman, persists for about 10 days, secreting both **oestrogens** and **progesterone**, before shrinking to form scar tissue (*corpus albicans*). The sudden rise in progesterone level increases the body temperature by ca. 0.5°C, which is sustained until the end of the cycle. However, if fertilization of the ovum/implantation *does* occur, the corpus luteum survives and continues to secrete steroids for two to three months, until the *placenta* takes over. The corpus luteum thus maintains the uterine endometrium during early pregnancy. The process of follicular maturation and ovulation is summarized in Figure 6.3.

The Uterine Cycle

The cyclic changes that occur in the endometrial lining prepare the uterus for possible fertilization and pregnancy. These changes, along with approximate times of their occurrence, may be summarized as follows:

1. *Day 1* of the menstrual cycle begins when the outer endometrial lining from the previous cycle is sloughed off, with loss of blood through the vagina (*menstrual phase*).
2. *Day 5*. Menstruation ceases, and **oestrogens** secreted by the developing follicles cause the endometrium to proliferate and to grow in thickness again (*follicular/proliferative phase*).
3. *Day 14* (mid-cycle). A surge in LH secretion occurs, followed 24–48 hours later by ovulation. **Progesterone** secreted by the corpus luteum stimulates the oestrogen-developed endometrium to become more vascular and to secrete mucus (*secretory/luteal phase*); this preparation is essential if implantation of a fertilized ovum is to occur.
4. *Day 28* (no fertilization). The corpus luteum regresses, hormonal support of the endometrium is lost, and menstruation begins again. The endometrium becomes

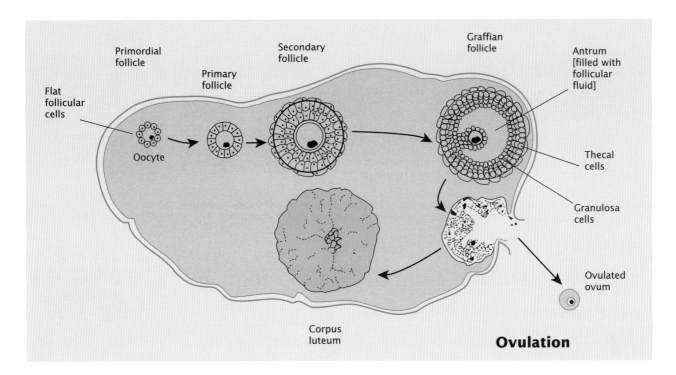

Figure 6.3. Sequential development of the ovarian follicle within the female ovary (not drawn to scale). During the *follicular phase*, a primordial follicle, consisting of an immature oocyte, protected by a flat layer of follicular cells, grows to form a primary, then a secondary follicle with surrounding layer of inner granulosa cells and outer thecal cells. A fluid-filled cavity (the antrum) forms around the oocyte. The mature ovarian follicle (Graafian) moves to the edge of the ovary and eventually ruptures (on about day 14 of the menstrual cycle) to release the ovum (ovulation). The follicular lining then collapses to form the corpus luteum (*luteal phase*) which eventually regresses if pregnancy does not occur. Only one follicle per cycle normally attains maturity and undergoes ovulation.

necrotic and breaks down due to shut-down of the spiral arteriolar blood supply.

These cyclical hormonal changes also alter the consistency and pH of the cervical mucus (clear, watery, stretchy, high pH at the time of ovulation to viscous, cellular, low pH after ovulation.

Hormonal Regulation of Menstrual Cycle

During the first 14 days of the cycle, the plasma FSH (and LH) levels slowly rise, which promotes ovarian follicle maturation and oestrogen secretion. The oestrogen enters the circulation and initially *inhibits* FSH secretion by a direct negative feedback effect on the pituitary (LH release is less affected) and hypothalamus (Figure 6.4), but at a certain maintained high threshold level, a switch to *positive feedback* occurs (see Chapter 1), and oestrogen now *stimulates a surge in LH* (lasting 24–48 hours), leading

ultimately to ovulation, corpus luteum formation and progesterone secretion. Progesterone also exerts a negative feedback effect on gonadotrophin secretion during the luteal phase.

As the LH level falls, the corpus luteum degenerates, normal negative feedback of oestrogen on the pituitary and hypothalamus is resumed, and menstruation follows when there is no longer enough oestrogen and progesterone available from the corpus luteum to maintain the endometrium; the cycle is then repeated.

The cyclic changes in plasma hormone levels that occur during the menstrual cycle are depicted in Figure 6.5.

☞ Granulosa cells also produce the peptide **inhibin** (on stimulation by FSH) which provides some negative feedback inhibition of FSH secretion during the follicular phase; (c.f. similar effect of testicular inhibin in males, p. 86–87). Inhibin is also produced by the corpus luteum during the luteal phase.

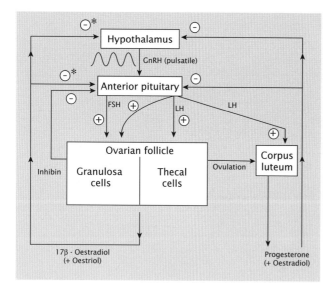

Figure 6.4. Control of female gonadal steroid production by the hypothalamus and anterior pituitary. Hypothalamic release of GnRH (pulsatile) stimulates the release of pituitary gonadotrophins LH and FSH which stimulate the thecal and granulosa cells of the ovarian follicle to produce oestrogens (17β-oestradiol and oestriol), and the corpus luteum (following ovulation) to produce progesterone (+ oestrogens). These hormones exert negative feedback effects on the hypothalamus and pituitary to control release of GnRH and LH; FSH release is regulated by a negative feedback loop involving the follicular peptide inhibin. [*A switch to *positive* feedback occurs at the time of ovulation, causing a surge in LH (and FSH) release].

Hormonal Changes During Pregnancy

If successful fertilization/uterine implantation of the ovum occurs (at about day 20), the *trophoblastic cells* surrounding the developing embryo secrete **human chorionic gonadotrophin (hCG)**, an LH-like glycoprotein hormone (composed of an α and a β subunit; see Chapter 2), which is detectable in the maternal urine within 9 days of conception and forms the basis of the common *pregnancy test* (see below). hCG maintains the corpus luteum (and therefore oestrogen/progesterone production) for about 9 weeks and so prevents further ovulation and menstruation, as well as maintaining the uterine lining. From about week 9, the *placenta* functions as an important endocrine gland and begins to secrete oestrogens (mainly **oestriol**, with **oestradiol** and **oestrone**) and progesterone, and continues to secrete large amounts of hCG. The hCG level eventually declines from its peak level in early pregnancy, to a maintained plateau after about week 16 (Figure 6.6), and the corpus luteum regresses. The exact functions of hCG during foetal development or the remaining pregnancy are uncertain,

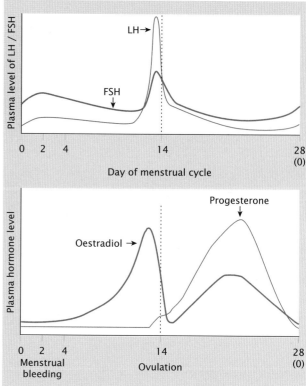

Figure 6.5. Changes in plasma levels of the pituitary gonadotrophins (LH and FSH) and ovarian hormones (17β-oestradiol and progesterone) during the 28 day female menstrual cycle. Note the steady rise in oestrogen level during the *follicular phase*, and the large surge in LH level at about mid-cycle, responsible for inducing ovulation; thereafter, the residual corpus luteum secretes progesterone (+ oestrogens) during the *luteal phase*, peaking at about day 22 (prior to onset of the next menstrual period). Note that in men, such cyclic fluctuations in plasma LH/FSH levels do not occur.

however it is thought to play an important role in stimulating the Leydig cells of the male foetal testes to produce **testosterone** and also in stimulating the foetal adrenal gland to produce the androgenic steroid precursor **dehydroepiandrosterone sulphate (DHEAS)** (utilized by the placenta to produce oestrogens).

Chorionic gonadotrophin (hCG) prepared from the urine of pregnant women (*Pregnyl; Profasi*, given by intramuscular injection) may be utilized for its LH-like activity to treat anovulatory infertility and also in the management of delayed male puberty or for stimulating descent of the testes in male children with *cryptorchidism*. A rare form of hCG-secreting brain tumour can cause *pseudoprecocious puberty* in boys.

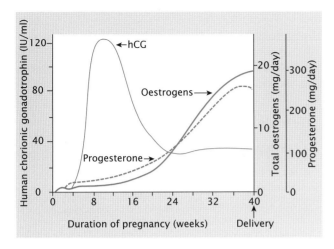

Figure 6.6. Maternal blood concentrations of oestrogens, progesterone and human chorionic gonadotrophin (hCG) during normal human pregnancy. After about week nine, the placenta takes over from the corpus luteum as the major source of oestrogens and progesterone.

From about the 5th week of pregnancy, the placenta also secretes **human chorionic somatomammotrophin (hCS)** (also called *human placental lactogen, hPL*), a 191 amino acid peptide, similar in structure to human GH and prolactin, as well as a range of other hypothalamic/pituitary-like peptides (e.g. GnRH and prolactin). Although large amounts of hCS are present in maternal blood, the exact role of this hormone in pregnancy is uncertain; however, it is believed to influence maternal carbohydrate and lipid metabolism to assure a constant supply of nutrients (particularly glucose) to the foetus. It may also exert some weak GH-like activity on foetal growth, and stimulate the partial development of breast tissue in preparation for lactation.

☞ A wide range of other proteins are also produced by placental tissue. In particular, **pregnancy-associated plasma protein A (PAPP-A)** and **pregnancy-specific beta 1-glycoprotein (SP-1)** have been isolated and studied in some detail, although the exact biological function of these peptides still remains uncertain. Circulating levels of hPL and SP-1 in the maternal serum (measured by radioimmunoassay) can be useful indicators of placental weight/function and foetal well-being during pregnancy. hCG, hPL and SP-1 can also be produced ectopically by certain adrenal or urinary tract carcinomas and may therefore be useful as diagnostic markers of these malignant tumours.

Relaxin is a small, two-chain polypeptide (53 amino acids) that is structurally similar to insulin and the IGF's (see Chapter 5). It is synthesized within the surviving corpus luteum of the ovary (and by the placenta) and is released into the maternal blood throughout pregnancy (it is also secreted by the male prostate gland and appears in seminal fluid). The main actions proposed for this peptide are to loosen the pubic ligaments and to soften ('ripen') and dilate the cervix in preparation for delivery. Although relaxin can act synergistically with progesterone to reduce spontaneous uterine contractions in some animal species, the current view is that this direct inhibitory action of relaxin on the myometrium may be of little importance in the regulation of uterine activity in human pregnancy. The possibility of using *recombinant human relaxin (rhRlx)* as a potential cervical softening agent applied intravaginally or intracervically prior to parturition is currently being evaluated.

SYNTHESIS OF STEROIDS BY THE MATERNAL FOETAL-PLACENTAL UNIT

Placental **progesterone** (synthesized in large quantities from maternal cholesterol, via *pregnenolone*) is utilized by the foetal adrenal gland to produce **cortisol** and **aldosterone**. It is also important in preventing uterine contractions during the pregnancy (and therefore premature expulsion of the foetus) and for preparing the mammary glands for eventual milk secretion.

Placental **oestrogens** serve an important function in stimulating the continued growth of the breast ductal system, and also stimulating the enlargement of the woman's external genitalia. In addition oestrogens cause relaxation of the pelvic ligaments, thereby facilitating the further expansion of the pregnant uterus. **Oestradiol** and **oestrone** are synthesized within the placenta from maternal and foetal *DHEAS*, whereas *oestriol* is formed from the hydroxylated precursor *(16-OH)-DHEAS*, derived from the foetal adrenal gland and liver (mainly) (Figure 6.7). The high levels of oestrogens exert a maintained negative feedback effect on the hypothalamus and pituitary during pregnancy, thereby preventing LH/FSH release, further follicle development and ovulation.

The Menopause

Between the ages of 45 to 55, menstruation in women normally becomes irregular and eventually ceases (the *menopause*). At this stage, very few functional primordial follicles are left within the ovaries. About 80% of women can then experience unpleasant post-menopausal symptoms that can be largely associated with the decline in oestrogen production. These include: *hot flushes of the skin, sweating, palpitations, increased irritability, anxiety, depression, vaginal atrophy* and the gradual development of *osteoporosis* (loss of bone mass and demineralization, with

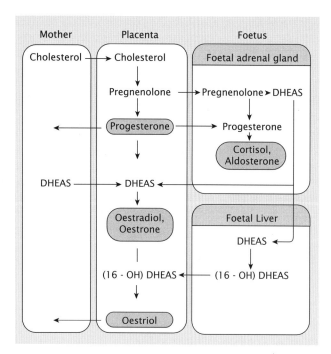

Figure 6.7. Synthesis of steroid hormones within the maternal foetal-placental unit. Progesterone is synthesized by the placenta from maternal cholesterol, which is then converted (via DHEAS) to oestrogens, oestradiol and oestrone. Progesterone also passes to the foetus, where it is converted to cortisol and aldosterone by the foetal adrenal gland. Foetal pregnenolone undergoes conversion to DHEAS in the adrenal and to (16-OH)-DHEAS in the foetal liver. Both DHEAS and (16-OH)-DHEAS are carried back to the placenta to produce oestrogens (principally oestriol). Placental progesterone and oestrogens enter the maternal circulation to affect uterine motility/growth and breast development.

increased risk of bone fractures, particularly of the spine and hip; see Chapter 7).

☞ Due to absence of hormonal negative feedback, plasma LH and FSH levels are high in post-menopausal women, although no cyclic variation is present. Follicular oestrogens are no longer secreted, but some oestrogen production can still occur through the peripheral conversion (aromatization) of ovarian or adrenal androgens; the main oestrogen becomes *oestrone* rather than *oestradiol* (see Figure 3.3).

Menotrophin (*Pergonal*), a highly purified preparation of gonadotrophins extracted from post-menopausal urine, may be given by intramuscular injection to stimulate follicular development and to induce ovulation in cases of infertility due to hypopituitarism; it may also be used to

treat hypogonadism due to lack of gonadotrophins in males. **Urofollitrophin** (*Metrodin*) containing purified menopausal FSH, may similarly be used to induce superovulation (multiple follicular growth) as part of an assisted conception, *in vitro* fertilization (IVF) technique.

Female Sex Hormones

OESTROGENS

The major oestrogenic steroid secreted by the ovary is **17β-oestradiol**, together with some **oestrone** (in chemical equilibrium) and **oestriol**. Oestrogens are also secreted by the corpus luteum, by the placenta during pregnancy, and in very small amounts by the adrenal cortex. Only 2% of circulating oestradiol exists as free hormone, the remainder being bound to plasma albumin (60%) or *sex hormone binding globulin (SHBG)* (38%) (c.f. testosterone p. 87); oestriol has a relatively low affinity for SHBG.

Oestrogens are necessary for normal development/maintenance of the female genital tract and the breasts.

The principal effects of oestrogenic hormones may be listed as follows:

1. *During puberty*, they stimulate the growth of the uterus, breasts and vagina, and control fat deposition and distribution in subcutaneous tissues, thereby determining the characteristic female figure. Like testosterone in the male, they are the primary cause of the 'growth spurt', closure of the epiphyses of the long bones and development of secondary sexual characteristics.

   ☞ Growth of pubic and underarm hair in the female is stimulated mainly by *adrenal androgen* secretion.

2. *In the adult*, oestrogens regulate events during the menstrual cycle (growth of endometrial lining), are important during pregnancy and lactation and contribute to the maintenance of sexual drive (*libido*) and female personality.

PROGESTOGENS

The main progestogen secreted by the ovary during the luteal phase is **progesterone**, responsible for the secretory changes in the uterine endometrium in preparation for pregnancy and (in cooperation with oestrogens) for stimulating the glandular development of the breasts in preparation for lactation. It also causes the cervical mucus to become thick and acidic, therefore less receptive to spermatozoa. Only 1–2% of circulating progesterone is unbound, with about 50% bound to albumin and the remainder to the corticosteroid-binding α_2-globulin *transcortin* (see Chapter 3).

During pregnancy, progesterone reduces the frequency of spontaneous contractions of the myometrium, which may be important if miscarriages are to be avoided. It has a weak negative feedback effect on the anterior pituitary and hypothalamus to control LH release.

Mechanism of Hormone Action. In common with other steroids, oestrogens and progesterone exert their effects by freely diffusing into target cells and combining with specific high affinity intracellular oestrogen or progesterone receptors respectively; these proteins belong to a superfamily of *ligand-activated transcription factors (LTFs)* which include receptors for thyroid hormone and the glucocorticoids. The resultant activated steroid-receptor complexes undergo conformational changes, loose chaperone *heat shock protein (Hsp-90;* see Chapter 3), dimerize, then bind to discrete nuclear DNA sequences and initiate (or suppress) the expression of specific genes i.e. synthesis of new mRNA and new proteins. The number of oestrogen and progesterone receptors in target tissues is controlled by prior oestrogen stimulation. Progesterone can also down-regulate its own receptor numbers. Abnormalities in the expression and function of oestrogen/progesterone receptors has been implicated in the development of certain disease states such as breast cancer, uterine fibroids or endometriosis (see below).

Clinical Disorders

Hyposecretion of oestrogens (*hypogonadism*) may result from the absence or inadequate function of the ovaries from birth. In this case, the normal female sex organs and secondary sexual characteristics do not develop, menstruation is absent (*primary amenorrhoea*), and closure of the epiphyses at the usual stage of adolescence does not occur. *Turner's syndrome* or *gonadal dysgenesis* (due to chromosomal abnormality: 45,XO) is the most common cause of congenital hypogonadism. This disorder (and related variants) where the defect lies in the gonad, is collectively termed *primary* or *hypergonadotrophic hypogonadism* (associated with high serum levels of LH and FSH). Premature ovarian failure (leading to *secondary amenorrhoea*) may also occur in some women under the age of 40, due to autoimmune disease. Alternatively, ovarian function may be defective due to lack of hypothalamic or pituitary hormones at puberty, referred to as *secondary* or *hypogonadotrophic hypogonadism.*

Lack of oestrogens due to premature removal of the ovaries in an adult woman, ultimately causes some regression of the sex organs and uterus and atrophy of the breasts, together with other symptoms characteristic of the menopause.

Hypersecretion of oestrogens may arise from ovarian granulosa-theca cell tumours (rare) and cause excessive oestrogenic effects, particularly on the uterus, where hypertrophy and irregular bleeding of the endometrium may occur.

ENDOMETRIOSIS

Endometriosis is a condition where endometrial tissue develops ectopically in the peritoneal cavity (usually close to the internal sex organs), most likely caused by retrograde menstruation along the fallopian tubes (peritoneal soiling). During each menstrual cycle, this ectopic tissue proliferates and degenerates like normal uterine endometrium, however, the ensuing haemorrhagic material accumulates in the abdomen usually causing irritation, severe cyclic abdominal or pelvic pain and development of *pelvic fibrosis.* Cyclical rectal bleeding or *haematuria* (blood in the urine) may also occur in some patients. If untreated, the condition may eventually result in infertility, due to fibrotic occlusion of the ovaries and fallopian tubes.

Treatment may involve surgery and/or drug therapy, depending on the severity of the disease. In mild cases, conservative surgical treatment is aimed at removing ectopic endometrial tissue and adhesions using a laparoscopic/laser ablation or laparotomy/microsurgical approach, in order to relieve symptoms and restore normal pelvic anatomy. In more severe cases, a complete removal of the uterus (*hysterectomy*) and ovaries (*bilateral oophorectomy*) may be necessary. Medical treatment is intended to provide symptomatic relief; some commonly used preparations include:

1. *Gonadotrophin release inhibitors:* **Danazol** *(Danol)* and **gestrinone** *(Dimetriose)* are synthetic progestogen derivatives (structurally related to testosterone), that inhibit gonadotrophin output at the pituitary and hypothalamic level, and thereby prevent ovulation; they also possess anti-progestogen and weak androgenic activity. These drugs are also useful for the treatment of gynaecomastia, benign breast tumours, cyclical breast pain (*mastalgia*), excessive menstrual bleeding (*menorrhagia*) and premenstrual syndrome, although some mild androgenic side effects (weight gain, hirsutism, greasy skin/acne, voice change) may follow from their use.

2. *The GnRH analogues:* **Buserelin, Goserelin, Leuprorelin,** or **Nafarelin** (see p. 98 and Chapter 2) may be given daily in the form of a nasal spray or by subcutaneous/intramuscular injection every month over 6 months to induce a hypo-oestrogenic state by suppressing pituitary gonadotrophin release. Menopausal-type side effects may, however, be induced including: *hot flushes, vaginal dryness* and *decreased libido.*

3. *Progestogens*: Synthetic progesterone derivatives such as **Norethisterone** (*Primolut N*), **Dydrogesterone** (*Duphaston*) or **Medroxyprogesterone** (*Provera*) may be given orally for 4–6 months or longer, or by intramuscular injection (*Depo-Provera*) to arrest endometrial growth and inhibit cyclic gonadotrophin release and ovulation.

Side effects *may include: irregular vaginal bleeding, weight gain, breast tenderness, headache and nausea.*

Some Clinical Uses of Oestrogens and Progestogens

A large variety of natural and synthetic oestrogens and progestogens are currently available for clinical use. The latter compounds, taken orally, are less prone to metabolism by the liver than the natural hormones, and are therefore preferred for therapeutic purposes.

CLINICAL USES OF OESTROGENS

Some commonly used oestrogens include: **17β-oestradiol, oestrone, oestriol, ethinyloestradiol, mestranol, dienoestrol** and **stilboestrol**.

Oestrogens may be used in:

1. *Hormone replacement therapy (HRT)*. Apart from their use in the treatment of various congenital hypo-ovarian conditions (e.g. *primary hypogonadism*) in young women (11–13 years), the most common use of oestrogens is in the amelioration of unpleasant menopausal symptoms (e.g. *hot flushes, night sweating, palpitations, headaches, vaginal dryness and atrophy*) due to the lack of natural oestrogens from the ovary. Such symptoms may also develop earlier, following surgical removal of the ovaries alone (*oophorectomy*) due to cancer, or together with the uterus (*hysterectomy*) in severe cases of endometriosis. Since natural oestrogens normally antagonize the Ca^{2+}-mobilizing effect of **parathyroid hormone** on bone (see Chapter 7), the provision of oestrogen supplements during *HRT* is important in the long-term, for preventing the development of post-menopausal osteoporosis and reducing bone fracture rate. HRT is also known to protect postmenopausal women from developing coronary heart disease (myocardial infarction and stroke) most likely by favourably affecting lipid/lipoprotein metabolism (oestrogens **increase** *high density lipoprotein [HDL]-cholesterol* and **decrease** potentially atherogenic *low density lipoprotein [LDL]-cholesterol* levels in the serum) and by also altering vascular blood flow (increasing arterial compliance); [some progestogens have the *opposite* effect on blood lipids, therefore could be reducing the beneficial effects of oestrogens on the lipid profile]. It has been suggested that HRT may be beneficial in women with existing cardiovascular disease.

Oestrogen-alone (unopposed) HRT is only appropriate for women who do not have an intact uterus (i.e. following hysterectomy); otherwise, a combined oestrogen/progestogen therapy is employed in order to reduce the risk of developing endometrial carcinoma (see below). In general, preparations using 'natural' oestrogens (oestradiol, oestrone or oestriol) rather than the more potent synthetic derivatives such as **ethinyloestradiol** or **mestranol** are preferred, always aiming for the lowest possible effective maintenance dose where possible.

Some commonly-used types of *oestrogen-only* preparation (listed in Table 6.1) include:

i) *Oral 'natural' oestrogen therapy:* Tablet preparations containing **oestradiol valerate, piperazine oestrone sulphate, oestriol**, or **conjugated equine oestrogens** are taken daily (from 28-tab. blister strips) on a continual basis.

ii) *Transdermal therapy* is advised for patients that cannot tolerate oral therapy, or where compliance is poor. This route avoids the first-pass metabolism of hormone by the liver, but is relatively expensive and can cause local skin irritation. Currently marketed self-adhesive oestrogen-only reservoir patches contain **17β-oestradiol** (*Estraderm TTS or MX [matrix patch]; Evorel; Fematrix*) and can be chosen to release between 25–100 μg hormone/24 hours; patches are placed on the trunk below the waistline (usually the buttocks, and never on or near the breasts) and replaced with a new patch after 3–4 days, on a continual basis. New '7 day' oestradiol patches, releasing about 50 μg hormone/24 hours are also now available (*FemSeven; Progynova TS*).

An oestrogen-containing gel (*Oestrogel*) with 0.06% **17β-oestradiol** was recently introduced, which can be rubbed into the skin of the arms, shoulders or inner thighs (but not the breasts or vaginal region) on a once-daily, continuous basis, as an alternative therapy for women with skin allergy to patches or where oral therapy is not preferred. Additional oral progestogen tablets can be co-prescribed where appropriate, for women with an intact uterus (see below). Skin contact with male partners should be avoided for an hour after application.

iii) *Implant therapy* may be used as an alternative to oral or transdermal therapy; implant preparations of **17β-oestradiol** are inserted subcutaneously (under clinical supervision) into the buttocks or abdomen every 4–8 months as necessary. An oral progestogen also needs to be taken for 10–14 days per cycle, if the uterus is intact.

iv) *Vaginal therapy.* Oestrogens e.g. **17β-oestradiol, oestriol, conjugated equine oestrogens** or **dienoestrol** (*Ortho Dienoestrol*), may also be applied topically as creams or in vaginal pessaries/modified-release tablets for short-term treatment of atrophic vaginal symptoms.

☞ Some vaginal creams can damage latex condoms and diaphragms.

Oestrogen	Type of preparation	Brand name (UK)
Oral 'natural' oestrogen therapy		
Oestradiol valerate (1–2 mg)	Tabs	Climaval
Oestradiol valerate (1–2 mg)	Tabs	Progynova Zumenon
Piperazine oestrone sulphate [Estropipate] (0.93 mg)	Tabs	Harmogen
Oestradiol, oestriol and oestrone mixture (0.27/1.4/0.6 mg)	Tabs	Hormonin
*Conjugated equine oestrogens (0.625–1.25 mg)	Tabs	Premarin
Transdermal therapy		
17-β-oestradiol (25–100 µg/24 hr)	Patches	Estraderm TTS/MX
17-β-oestradiol (25–75 µg/24 hr)	Patches	Evorel
17-β-oestradiol (40–80 µg/24 hr)	Patches	Fematrix
17-β-oestradiol (37.5–75 µg/24 hr)	Patches	Menorest
17-β-oestradiol (0.06%)	Gel	Oestrogel
Vaginal therapy		
Oestriol	Vaginal cream/pessary	Ortho-Gynest
Oestriol	Vaginal cream	Ovestin
Conjugated oestrogens	Vaginal cream	Premarin
Dienoestrol	Vaginal cream	Ortho-Dienoestrol
17-β-oestradiol	Vaginal tabs	Vagifem
17-β-oestradiol	Vaginal ring	Estring

* Conjugated oestrogens (derived from pregnant mare urine) consist of a mixture of **sodium oestrone sulphate** (ca. 60%) and **sodium equilin sulphate** (ca. 30%) (a natural equine oestrogen).

Table 6.1. Some examples of currently available preparations used for unopposed (oestrogen-only) hormone replacement therapy (HRT) for women without an intact uterus; [from *MIMS, June 1997*].

An impregnated silastic vaginal ring is also now available (*Estring*) which releases a constant amount (about 7.5 mg) of **17β-oestradiol hemihydrate** directly into the vagina every 24 hours; minimal systemic absorption of oestradiol takes place. It is worn continuously and replaced every three months; therapy may continue for up to two years. Regular examination of patients (every 3–6 months) is necessary to assess the need to continue treatment.

2. *Treatment of androgen-dependent prostatic cancer*
Administration of oestrogens, by altering the hormonal environment, may be used to limit the stimulatory effects of androgens on prostatic androgen-dependent malignant cells in men. The synthetic non-steroidal oestrogen **stilboestrol** may be given orally, although *feminization, testicular atrophy, impotence* and *breast growth (gynaecomastia)* may occur as side effects. In view of

these undesirable actions, administration of potent synthetic GnRH agonists such as **buserelin** (*Suprecur*), **goserelin** (*Zoladex*) or **leuprorelin** (*Prostap SR*), has become more popular for suppressing androgenic activity in treatment of advanced prostatic carcinoma. The long-term (non-pulsatile) administration of these agents (by nasal spray or by subcutaneous/intramuscular (depot) injection), produces a down-regulation of pituitary GnRH receptors, and an ultimate decrease in gonadotrophin and androgen secretion (see Chapter 2). Some initial *stimulation* ('flare') of tumour activity may occur before effective gonadotrophin inhibition is established; this can be controlled by treatment with an anti-androgen (e.g. **Flutamide**; see above, p. 89).

3. *Postcoital oral contraception (the 'morning after' pill)*
Pregnancy can be effectively prevented by short-term administration of a high dose of oestrogen in combination with a progestogen; (the mode of action is most likely to prevent implantation). The only preparation currently licensed in the UK is *Schering PC4* which consists of four tablets, containing 50 µg of **ethinyloestradiol** and 0.5 mg of the progestogen **norgestrel** (equivalent to 0.25 mg of the active isomer **levonorgestrel**). Treatment begun within 72 hours of unprotected intercourse (two tablets taken as soon as possible, followed by a further two after 12 hours), is reported to be at least 98% effective; some unpleasant *side effects* may however develop, associated with the high oestrogen content e.g. *nausea, vomiting,* (affecting absorbtion), *headache, dizziness* and *breast tenderness*; the menstrual pattern may also be temporarily disturbed. If conception does occur, it is considered unlikely that foetal development would be adversely affected by the PC4 hormone administration over the recommended period. Patients should however, be carefully examined for possible ectopic (tubal) pregnancy.

☞ In the USA, **stilboestrol** (called *diethylstilbestrol [DES]*, 25 mg tablets, twice daily for 5 days) may be given for emergency post-coital contraception, beginning within 72 hours of intercourse.

Oestrogen Antagonists. **Clomiphene** *(Clomid)* is an anti-oestrogenic drug which competes with oestrogens for cytoplasmic oestrogen receptors, but has little or no intrinsic oestrogenic activity; it therefore prevents the normal hormonal negative feedback inhibition on the hypothalamus and anterior pituitary, and induces a rise in GnRH and LH/FSH secretion (provided the hypothalamus and pituitary are functioning correctly). This drug is therefore used to stimulate ovulation in women that are infertile, although hyperovulation and multiple pregnancies may commonly occur.

Tamoxifen *(Tamofen; Nolvadex-D)* is a similarly-acting anti-oestrogen which is used to treat anovulatory infertility and has now become the treatment of choice for the treatment of advanced oestrogen-dependent breast tumours in women; (also **toremifene** (*Fareston*)). The potential use of tamoxifen for *preventing* the development of breast tumours in women considered to be at high risk (with positive family history) is currently being evaluated in the USA.

Side effects associated with the use of anti-oestrogens include *hot flushes, vaginal bleeding, abdominal discomfort, dizziness* and *visual disturbances*. Recent evidence also indicates a small but significant risk of developing *endometrial cancer* after long-term (>2 years) tamoxifen treatment.

Aromatase Inhibitors. **Aminoglutethimide** *(Orimeten)* is a potent (type II) aromatase enzyme inhibitor that is used for the management of advanced oestrogen-dependent breast cancer in post-menopausal or oophorectomized women (particularly in patients who have become resistant to tamoxifen), and also as a palliative treatment for advanced prostatic carcinoma in men. It blocks several cytochrome P-450 mediated steroid hydroxylation steps, particularly those involved in the adrenal conversion of *cholesterol* to *pregnenolone* (see Figure 3.3), as well as the peripheral aromatization of androgens to oestrogens (in fat, muscle and liver cells). Modern treatment schedules utilize lower daily doses of the inhibitor (250–500 mg) together with a replacement dose of corticosteroid (e.g. cortisone) in an attempt to avoid complicating side effects (e.g. drowsiness, dermatitis, blood disorders); the therapy is often referred to as *'medical adrenalectomy'* (replacing bilateral surgical adrenalectomy).

Aminoglutethimide is also used for the medical treatment of *Cushing's syndrome* (Chapter 3).

More specific (type I) aromatase inhibitors, **formestane** (*Lentaron*, given by deep intramuscular injection), **letrozole** (*Femara*) or **anastrozole** (*Arimidex*, both given orally) are also available for treatment of advanced post-menopausal breast carcinoma; unlike aminoglutethimide, these agents have no effect on adrenocortical steroid synthesis. Irritation at the injection site (formestane), hot flushes, sweating, vaginal dryness, thinning of the hair and lethargy/drowsiness may occur as side effects. Aromatase inhibitors are not indicated for use as suppressants of oestrogen synthesis in *pre*menopausal breast cancer patients.

CLINICAL USES OF PROGESTOGENS

Several orally-active progestogens are also available; these include: **Norethisterone, norgestrel, levonorgestrel, ethynodiol diacetate, medroxyprogesterone,** or the newer derivatives: **gestodene, desogestrel, norgestimate** and **dydrogesterone**.

Progestogens are mainly used in:

1. *Control of uterine bleeding and menstrual disturbances*
This includes control of painful *(dysmenorrhoea)* or excessively heavy menstruation *(menorrhagia)* and premenstrual syndrome; also in the treatment of endometriosis, and for postponement of menstruation.

2. *Oral contraception*
The principal use of progestogens alone is in the form of the oral progestogen-only contraceptive pill (POC) or *'mini-pill'*. Taken daily (starting from the first day of the period and throughout), the POC is rather less reliable in preventing pregnancy than the 'combined' contraceptive pill described below. The major contraceptive action is probably due to the unfavourable changes produced in the endometrium (making implantation less likely) and cervical mucus (becoming thick, sticky and hostile to sperm), coupled with a weak (and variable) negative feedback inhibition of LH release and ovulation; fallopian tube motility (affecting ovum transport) may also be reduced. In some women, administration of POCs can completely suppress gonadotrophin secretion and ovulation, resulting in amenorrhoea (absent menstruation); in others, ovulation and menstrual cycles occur in a near normal fashion. Some decrease in motility of the fallopian tubes (important for successful fertilization) may also be induced.

3. *Depot injections and capsule implants*
Depot (slow release) preparations of progestogens can also be used for more long-term contraception, particularly in patients unable to tolerate other contraceptives, or where compliance is poor; they are given either by deep intramuscular injection at 2–3 monthly intervals e.g. **Medroxyprogesterone acetate** *(Depo-Provera)* or **norethisterone enanthate** *(Noristerat)*, or subdermally as an implant into the upper part of a non-dominant arm (**levonorgestrel**; *Norplant*), the latter giving highly effective contraceptive protection for up to 5 years (expensive!). Unlike depot injections, fertility may return quite rapidly (within 48 hours) after removal of the implants.

☞ Depot progestogens may also be used in breast/endometrial cancer therapy.

A novel form of intrauterine device (IUD; see below) that releases **levonorgestrel** into the uterine cavity (20 mg/24 hrs, over 3 years) has recently been introduced (*Mirena*) (see below).

Side effects associated with the use of POCs or other progestogen-only preparations are relatively minor and include: *irregular menstrual bleeding/spotting,* (particularly on first starting use) due to the continued progestogen stimulation of the endometrium, *headache, nausea, depression, acne, fluid retention (weight gain), hypertension, breast discomfort* and *possible persistence of infertility* for several months after withdrawal of treatment.

In view of the absence of serious side effects, POCs are considered more suitable for use than the combined pill in older women (over 35 years), heavy smokers, those with a history of thromboembolism or hypertension, or where oestrogens are generally not advised (e.g. diabetic women; see Chapter 5). The small doses of progestogen used causes minimal disruption of lipid or carbohydrate metabolism. There is a weak risk of ectopic pregnancy developing in patients that do become pregnant whilst taking a POC (due to decreased tubal motility).

Progestogens in combination with oestrogens are mainly used in:

1. *Combined oestrogen/progestogen preparations for oral contraception (COCs)*
Low dose synthetic oestrogen/progestogen combinations *(the 'pill')* are regarded as very effective, easy to use and relatively safe contraceptives. The oestrogen content (typically between 20–50 µM) suppresses ovulation by inhibiting LH/FSH release, thereby mimicking the normal negative feedback effect of the natural oestrogens at the pituitary and hypothalamic level; the progestogen content induces the cervical mucus to become thick and more resistant to sperm penetration, and the endometrium to become thin and inadequately developed for implantation. Three types of preparation are currently available:

Monophasic combination tablets contain a single synthetic oestrogen/progestogen dose combination, and are taken daily (from a 'blister' pack) starting on the first or fifth day of menstruation, for 21 days followed by a 7-day interval of dummy (placebo) tablets (or pill-free days) during which the sudden removal of progestogen initiates *'withdrawal menstruation'* (the latter may be psychologically reassuring to some women, that pregnancy has indeed been prevented); the cycle is then repeated. It is essential that the tablets are taken at the same time each day, as their effectiveness can fall if they are taken late or missed (i.e. taken more than 12 hours late). Effectiveness can also be reduced if they are taken in combination with other drugs that influence oestrogen/progestogen metabolism (e.g. *barbiturates, phenytoin, phenylbutazone, rifampicin, griseofulvin*) or certain broad-spectrum antibiotics that affect the gastrointestinal flora (*ampicillin* and *tetracyclines*).

Biphasic or triphasic combination tablets contain oestrogen/progestogen combination doses that vary throughout the cycle; (this may be more suitable for some women, than the monophasic preparations). The tablets are started on day 1 or day 5 of a period and must be taken in the correct order to be effective (1 daily for 21 days, then 7 tablet-free [or placebo] days).

☞ Combined oral contraceptive therapy, by providing a regular withdrawal bleed, may also be useful for some women who normally suffer from excessively heavy, painful or irregular periods.

Mild side effects of the combined pills are mostly related to the oestrogen content and may include: *nausea, vomiting, weight gain* (due to Na^+/fluid retention), *mild hypertension, breast tenderness, leg pains, cramps, loss of libido, depression* (may counteract effect of anti-depressant drugs), *migraine-type headache, visual disturbances, decreased tolerance to contact lenses, increased skin pigmentation* and *impairment of glucose tolerance* (important for diabetic patients).

☞ The health risks associated with unwanted pregnancy resulting from unprotected intercourse or less reliable methods of contraception are considered to be much greater than those of combined pill therapy, particularly in less developed countries.

In very rare cases: *venous thromboembolism* (oestrogens increase blood coagulation), *cerebral haemorrhage/embolism/stroke, myocardial infarction* (particularly in heavy smokers over 35 years of age) or *breast/cervical cancer* can occur: (the suppression of the ovarian cycle by the oral contraceptives actually *reduces* the risk of developing ovarian or endometrial cancer). Withdrawal of treatment may cause amenorrhoea in some patients; however, this should not last longer than a few months. It is advisable to discontinue combined pill therapy prior to any major surgery, in order to avoid the risk of thromboembolism.

The two synthetic oestrogens commonly used for oral contraception are **ethinyloestradiol** and **mestranol**. Some currently available preparations are listed in Table 6.2.

☞ A warning issued to doctors in October 1995 by the UK committee on safety of medicines, indicated that the use of the newer generation combined contraceptive pills containing the progestogens **desogestrel** or **gestodene** was associated with a twofold greater risk of developing thromboembolisms compared with formulations containing the androgenic progestogens **levonorgestrel** or **norethisterone**. Prescribers were advised to switch their patients to alternative pills where possible, or where this was not acceptable, to fully explain the increased health risks to patients before continuing treatment. Affected women also needed to be assured that the risk of suffering thrombosis from an unplanned pregnancy was still considered to be greater than that posed by taking COCs.

2. *Oestrogen/progestogen preparations for postmenopausal HRT*
Since prolonged (>1 year) unopposed exposure to oestrogens in postmenopausal women with an intact uterus can lead to excessive endometrial stimulation (hyperplasia) and possible endometrial cancer, it is important to include a progestogen for the last 10–14 days of every treatment cycle, in addition to the oestrogen, as part of the HRT protocol. Synthetic progestogens such as **levonorgestrel, norethisterone, medroxyprogesterone** or **norgestrel** are used, rather than progesterone itself, which is metabolised too quickly to be effective (plasma half-life ca. 5 min). 'Combined' HRT is usually begun as soon as possible after onset of the menopause, or in the 'peri-menopausal' phase (when periods are becoming irregular) and may involve a wide range of hormone preparations, depending on individual requirements, tolerance and preference. The usual therapy period is between 18 months–5 years, although some women persist with HRT for longer periods of time (up to 10 years or more); the possible increased risk of developing breast cancer following long-term HRT is still controversial.

Examples of some combined HRT preparations (for women with an intact uterus) containing **oestradiol valerate** or **conjugated equine oestrogens** with either **norethisterone, levonorgestrel, dydrogesterone**, or **medroxyprogesterone** are listed in Table 6.3.

In sequential therapy, tablets are usually taken daily (from 28 tab. blister packs) starting with 1 oestrogen-containing tablet/day for up to 16 days, followed by 1 combined oestrogen/progestogen-containing tablet/day for the remaining 12 days (repeated on a monthly cyclical basis) with a regular withdrawal bleed occurring at the end of each cycle; this may, however be unacceptable to many menopausal women receiving HRT for the first time. Indeed, poor patient compliance in HRT is a substantial problem.

In women of 54 years of age (or at least 1 year after the last period), *continuous combined HRT* is recommended, in which daily doses of oestrogen and progestogen are taken over a 25 day regimen, with no cyclical withdrawal bleed.

Transdermal reservoir patches releasing **17β-oestradiol** (50 µg/24 hr) and **norethisterone** (250 µg/24 hr) (*Estracombi*) may also be used, applied to the skin below the waistline and replaced every 3–4 days using a different site; oestrogen-only patches are applied for 2 weeks, followed by combined patches for 2 weeks on a cyclical basis. A similar matrix patch formulation (*Nuvelle TS*) releasing 80 µg **oestradiol**/24 h (twice weekly for 2 weeks) followed by a combined patch (delivering 50 µg **oestradiol** plus 20 µg **levonorgestrel**/24 h, twice weekly for next 2 weeks) has also recently been introduced.

Side effects of combined HRT are similar (though less severe) to those described above for combined oral contraceptives.

Oestrogen	Progestogen	Brand name (UK)
Combined (monophasic) type		
Ethinyloestradiol (30 μg)	Norethisterone (1.5 mg)	Loestrin 30
Ethinyloestradiol (30 μg)	Levonorgestrel (0.15 mg)	Microgynon 30
Ethinyloestradiol (30 μg)	Gestodene (75 μg)	Femodene ED*
Mestranol (50 μg)	Norethisterone (1 mg)	Norinyl-1
Biphasic/triphasic type		
Ethinyloestradiol (35/35 μg)	Norethisterone (0.5/1 mg)	BiNovum
Ethinyloestradiol (30/40/30 μg)	Gestodene (50/70/100 μg)	Triadene
Ethinyloestradiol (30/40/30 μg)	Levonorgestrel (50/75/125 μg)	Logynon ED*
Progestogen only		
—	Ethynodiol diacetate(0.5 mg)	Femulen
—	Levonorgestrel (30 μg)	Norgeston
—	Norethisterone (0.35 mg)	Noriday

*28 ED ('everyday' packs) also contain 7 inert lactose tablets.

[Compiled from *MIMS*, June 1997].

§ Oral contraceptive preparations marketed in the USA consist of various combinations of oestrogenic compounds (*ethinyloestradiol* or *mestranol*) together with synthetic progestogens (*norethindrone, norgestrel, levonorgestrel, norgestimate desogestrel* or *ethynodiol diacetate*). The brand names include:
Brevicon, Demulen, Levlen, Lo-Ovral, Modicon, Nelova, Norinyl, Nordette, Ortho-Cept, Ortho-Cyclen, Ortho-Novum, Ortho-Tricyclen, Ovcon, Ovral, Tri-Levlen, Tri Norinyl and *Triphasil*.

Table 6.2. Some examples of currently available oral contraceptive preparations§.

Adjuctive progestogens. Progestogen-only tablets containing **Norethisterone** (*Micronor-HRT*) or **dydrogesterone** (*Duphaston-HRT*) can be given daily with oestrogen-alone preparations on a cyclical or continuous basis, whenever a combined HRT approach is required.

Tibolone (*Livial*) is a synthetic hormone derivative that possesses both oestrogenic and progestogenic (as well as weak androgenic) activity, and has therefore been recently introduced in HRT for short-term treatment of vasomotor symptoms resulting from the menopause, without the need for cyclical progestogen supplements; the 'withdrawal bleeding' that occurs with other combination preparations is thus avoided. It is more costly than other forms of treatment, and some androgenic side effects (hirsutism) may develop with its use. It is not recommended for long-term protection against osteoporosis or for treatment of atrophic vaginitis.

Progestogen Antagonist

Mifepristone (*Mifegyne; RU 486*) competes with progesterone for binding to cytoplasmic progesterone receptors and thereby acts as a progestogen antagonist. It is given orally (followed in 36–48 hours by an intra-vaginal prostaglandin pessary [**Gemeprost**], under careful medical supervision) as an abortifacient agent in obstetrics to terminate intra-uterine pregnancies of up to 63 days of gestation (ca. 85% effective). Severe vaginal bleeding, nausea, vomiting and incomplete abortion may occur as side effects.

Intrauterine Devices (IUDs)

These have been use in family planning for many years, and are popular with women who require a highly effective

Oestrogen	Progestogen	Brand name (UK)
Tablets (sequential therapy)		
Oestradiol valerate (1–2 mg)	Norethisterone (1 mg)	Climagest
Oestradiol valerate (2 mg)	Levonorgestrel (75 µg)	Nuvelle
Oestradiol valerate (2 mg)	Norgestrel (500 µg)	Cyclo-Progynova
Oestradiol valerate (2 mg)	Dydrogesterone (10 mg)	Femoston 2/10
Conjugated equine oestrogens (0.625–1.25 mg)	Norgestrel (150 µg)	Prempak-C
Oestradiol (2 mg) + Oestriol (1 mg)	Norethisterone (1 mg)	Trisequens
Tablets (Continuous therapy)		
Oestradiol valerate (2 mg)	Norethisterone (0.7/1 mg)	Climesse
		Kliofem
Conjugated oestrogens (0.625 mg)	Medroxy-progesterone (5 mg)	Premique
Transdermal patches		
17-β-oestradiol (50 µg/24 hr)	Norethisterone (250 µg/24 hr)	Estracombi
17-β-oestradiol (50 µg/24 hr)	Norethisterone (1 mg)	Estrapak (patches and tabs)
17-β-oestradiol (80/50 µg/24 hr)	Levonorgestrel (20 µg)	Nuvelle TS (matrix patches)

[Compiled from *MIMS*, June 1997].

Table 6.3. Some examples of currently available preparations used for combined hormone replacement therapy (HRT) for women with an intact uterus.

and continuous mode of contraception, but do not wish to use hormonal methods. Nowadays, they all consist of a copper wire wound onto an inert polythene T-shaped carrier (with a thread attached to the base of the stem for removal) that is inserted into the uterus under medical supervision, and changed every 3–5 years as the Cu is gradually eluted; [devices fitted in women over 40 years may be left in place until the menopause]. The Cu wire has a silver core to avoid fragmentation (ca. 200–350 mm² Cu surface is exposed). Their exact mode of action in preventing conception is still unclear, but most probably involves the induction of a local inflammatory response and alteration in enzyme activity within the uterus that interferes with egg implantation, coupled with a direct spermicidal effect of the Cu ions.

Side effects associated with the use of IUDs include: *abnormal uterine bleeding and pain, heavy menstruation* (menorrhagia), development of *pelvic inflammatory disease* (*PID*; due to transmitted infection) or more rarely: risk of *ectopic pregnancy, uterine/cervical perforation, displacement or expulsion of the IUD from the uterus, Cu allergy and epileptic*

attack on insertion. The devices should be removed immediately if accidental pregnancy occurs.

Some currently available IUDs in the UK include:

the *Multiload Cu 375, Novagard, Ortho-gyne T/380 Slimline* and the *Nova-T*.

☞ The only Cu-containing IUDs presently marketed in the USA are the *Paragard T-380A* intrauterine copper contraceptive and the *Lippes Loop Double-S* intrauterine device.

Progestogen-releasing IUD

A new form of intrauterine contraceptive device is now available (*Mirena*), consisting of a plastic T-shaped carrier frame impregnated with a *levonorgestrel/silastic* mixture, designed to release 20 µg of hormone/24 hr into the uterine cavity. Once fitted, it is effective in preventing conception for up to 3 years, mainly due to a potent local endometrial suppression, although suppression of ovulation may also occur in some women. Rapid return of fertility occurs after removal. It is particularly recommended for women with heavy menstrual periods or those who require long-term contraception, but are unable or unwilling to take oral contraceptives. Intrauterine release of levonorgestrel is also being considered as an alternative way of adding a progestogen component to continuous HRT regimens.

Side effects (particularly during the first month of use) include: *changes in menstrual pattern, headache, acne,* and *nausea-* declining with prolonged use. The risk of developing PID or ectopic pregnancy, is significantly less than that associated with Cu-containing IUDs.

Pregnancy Testing

Several varieties of home pregnancy testing kit are readily available from retail pharmacy outlets, which are relatively quick (3–5 min), easy to use and highly accurate (*e.g. Clearblue One Step; First response; Discover Today*). All are based on the detection of **human chorionic gonadotrophin (hCG)** in a fresh (ideally first of the day) urine sample, by means of a sensitive indicator kit; a change in colour of the indicator generally shows a positive result. The test is normally performed on the day a period is due, with a re-test after 3 days to confirm a negative result.

Home ovulation prediction tests (*First Response; Clear Plan One Step*) can also be performed on urine samples to detect the pre-ovulatory surge in LH that occurs during the menstrual cycle, and therefore help to pinpoint the most fertile period for conception. They are not meant to be used as a means of contraception. ■

Review Questions

Question 1:   State the location and main functions of the gonads.

Question 2:   Define the terms androgen, oestrogen, progestogen. Give examples of the naturally secreted hormones of each group.

Question 3:   Outline the structure and histology of the testes.

Question 4:   State from which testicular cells testosterone is secreted.

Question 5:   Describe the mechanisms controlling testosterone release.

Question 6:   Summarize the main effects of testosterone:
(a) in the foetus,
(b) during puberty,
(c) in the adult.

Question 7:   What is the function of müllerian inhibiting substance (MIS) during male foetal development?

Question 8:   Outline how testosterone exerts its effects via intracellular receptors.

Question 9:   Explain the importance of 5α-dihydrotestosterone (DHT) in mediating the actions of testosterone in some tissues; how is the conversion of testosterone to DHT brought out?

Question 10:   Describe the conditions that may lead to hyposecretion or hypofunction of testosterone, and explain their consequences.

Question 11:   Describe (giving named drug examples) the clinical uses for androgens:
(a) in replacement therapy,
(b) as protein anabolic agents,
(c) in breast/cervical cancer treatment.

Question 12:   What general side effects would you associate with androgen therapy?

Question 13:   Give examples of anti-androgenic compounds and their uses/side effects.

Question 14:   What is benign prostatic hyperplasia (BPH)? How may this condition be treated?

Question 15:   Outline the structure of the ovaries and ovarian follicles.

Question 16:   Explain the processes of:
(a) follicular maturation under influence of LH/FSH,
(b) ovulation (after LH surge).

Question 17:   State from which ovarian cells oestrogens and progesterone are secreted.

Question 18:   Describe the cyclic changes occurring in the endometrium during the menstrual cycle.

Question 19:   Describe the cyclic hormonal changes that occur (a) during the menstrual cycle (b) during pregnancy.

Question 20:   Explain the significance of human chorionic gonadotrophin (hCG) as the basis of the pregnancy test.

Question 21:   What is the source and proposed role of relaxin during pregnancy?

Question 22:   Outline the synthetic pathways for steroid synthesis by the maternal foetal-placental unit.

Question 23:   Give the major symptoms that may be associated with the female menopause.

Question 24:   Summarize the main effects of oestrogens (a) during puberty, (b) in the adult.

Question 25:   Summarize the main effects of progesterone (a) during the menstrual cycle, (b) during pregnancy.

Question 26:   Outline how oestrogens and progestogens exert their biological effects via intracellular receptors.

Question 27:   Describe the conditions leading to hyposecretion and hypersecretion of oestrogens and their consequences.

Question 28:   Describe the condition of endometriosis and its treatment.

Question 29:   Give (with named examples) some clinical uses of oestrogens and progestogens including:

Oestrogen-only preparations: *for (a) hormone replacement therapy (HRT).*
(b) treatment of prostatic cancer, (c) post-coital contraception;
Progestogen-only preparations: *for (a) treatment of menstrual disturbances.*
(b) oral contraception (POCs), (c) depot injections/implants;
Combined preparations: *for (a) oral contraception (COCs). (b) HRT.*

Question 30: *Give examples of oestrogen and progestogen antagonists and their clinical uses.*

Question 31: *What are aromatase inhibitors? How are these drugs used clinically?*

Question 32: *Describe the use of combined oestrogen/progestogen preparations for oral contraception; give examples of the types of preparation currently available and explain their mode of action.*

Question 33: *List the side effects associated with the use of POCs and combined oral contraceptive pills.*

Question 34: *Explain the nature and mode of action of intrauterine devices (IUD's), and list the side effects associated with their use.*

Clinical Case Studies

Patient 1

An 18 year old boy was brought to the clinic with a history of bifrontal headaches and blurred vision of three months duration. There was no previous medical illness. Clinical examination revealed a lack of secondary sex characteristics (sparse axillary and pubic hair, absence of beard/moustache and chest hair, decreased muscle mass). Examination of the eyes revealed papilloedema (swollen discs). The remainder of the clinical examination was unremarkable. An MRI (magnetic resonance image) scan of the hypothalamic-pituitary area showed the presence of a suprasellar mass.

Laboratory investigation revealed a normal FBC, urinalysis and blood chemistry. Hormonal studies gave a serum testosterone level of 25 ng/dl (normal male 300–1110 ng/dl), an LH level of 3 mIU/ml (normal 4–30 mIU/ml) and an FSH level of 2 mIU/ml (normal 4–30 mIU/ml). Serum prolactin was normal.

Question 1: *What is the most likely cause of this patient's problem?*

Question 2: *How is the condition diagnosed?*

Question 3: *What is the recommended treatment?*

Answer 1: This patient has a low testosterone level, low-normal gonadotrophin levels and a lack of secondary sexual characteristics, suggestive of *hypogonadotrophic hypogonadism (secondary hypogonadism)*. Broadly, hypogonadism is classified as primary (where the defect lies in the gonads) or secondary (where the defect is in the pituitary or hypothalamus). The former is also known as *hypergonadotropic hypogonadism*.

Answer 2: Diagnosis of hypogonadism is made by documentation of low gonadal sex steroid hormone levels. Clinically, the signs of secondary sexual maturation may be lacking. Whether the defect is primary or secondary, the sex steroid levels will be characteristically low. However in *secondary hypogonadism*, treatment with gonadotrophins should raise the sex steroid level. A decrease in circulating testosterone normally results in escape of the pituitary/hypothalamic axis from negative feedback, leading to a rise in LH and FSH levels. Absence of such a rise, as in this case, points to a defect in the hypothalamo-pituitary region. Blurred vision and *papilloedema* (swelling of the optic disc) also suggests a hypothalamic/pituitary lesion that is compressing the optic chiasm. An alternative cause of the patient's hypogonadotropic hypogonadism i.e. a prolactin-secreting pituitary adenoma (causing hyperprolactinaemia) is ruled out by the normal serum prolactin levels.

Answer 3: Patients with secondary hypogonadism can be treated with replacement androgens and/or gonadotrophins (*Menotrophin: human menopausal gonadotrophins [hMG], LH/FSH,* by intramuscular injection) or *pulsatile GnRH* (subcutaneously via portable pump, provided the pituitary gland is normal) or intramuscular *human chorionic gonadotrophin (hCG; LH-like)/ hMG* combination treatment. However, when the defect is at the testicular level, replacement androgens are the only available form of treatment, since the testes would be incapable of responding to administered gonadotrophins.

A diagnosis of acquired hypogonadism secondary to *craniopharyngioma* was made, and the patient underwent successful surgical (trans-sphenoidal) resection of the pituitary mass. He was subsequently placed on androgen replacement therapy (three-weekly intramuscular injections of *testosterone enanthate*) to promote normal development of sexual characteristics and muscle mass, with additional later treatment with *menotrophin* to establish fertility.

Patient 2

A 32 year old female was referred to the hospital Endocrinology Department for evaluation of amenorrhoea (absent menstruation). The patient was in good health until eight months previous, when she started noticing scanty menstruation followed by complete cessation two months later. One year earlier, she had started experiencing occasional episodes of hot flushes and anxiety. This had become more pronounced in the last four months. The patient had been married for the past eight years, and had had two successful pregnancies in this time, but reported loss of libido in the past one year. She had no other medical history. Physical examination revealed fine wrinkles under the eyes, and a thin dry skin; the remainder of the examination was normal.

Laboratory data indicated a serum oestradiol level of 18 pg/ml (normal >25 pg/ml) with serum levels of LH and FSH at 57 mIU/ml and 40 mIU/ml respectively (normal female 4–30 mIU/ml for both LH and FSH). Thyroid hormone levels were normal, and she did not test positive for thyroid antibodies; serum prolactin measurement also revealed a normal level. There was no evidence of adrenal insufficiency or diabetes mellitus.

Question 1: *Based upon the patient's history, physical examination and laboratory data, what is the most likely diagnosis of her condition?*

Question 2: *How may this condition arise?*

Question 3: *What would be the recommended therapy for this patient?*

Answer 1: This case is characterized by a low oestrogen level, associated with increased levels of gonadotrophins (*hypergonadotropic hypogonadism*), suggesting the ovaries as the most likely target of dysfunction. Usually, this hormonal pattern, coupled with amenorrhoea, hot flushes of the skin and anxiety, is only seen at the time of the menopause.

Answer 2: The patient is most likely suffering from a *premature ovarian failure (POF)*, leading to *secondary amenorrhoea;* [this refers to individuals who once menstruated, but subsequently stopped menstruating; *primary amenorrhoea* refers to patients who have never menstruated]. In about 20% of cases of POF, the condition is due to specific autoimmune disease, accompanied by the presence of serum antiovarian antibodies (causing accelerated oocyte degeneration) or it may be part of a polyglandular autoimmune syndrome, where the thyroid, adrenal glands and pancreas are also affected. Most commonly, abnormal thyroid function may be detected, hence the need to check thyroid hormone levels and thyroid antibodies. Classically, ovarian failure precedes adrenal failure, and a case can be made for continuing adrenal surveillance.

Answer 3: Ovulation can sometimes be temporarily restored with oral corticosteroid treatment however, in general the return of normal menses (and fertility) is unlikely. In this case, the clinical symptoms of hypogonadism and the long-term risk of osteoporosis warrant hormone replacement therapy (HRT). Since the uterus is intact, oestrogens should be cycled with progestogens to induce regular withdrawal menstruation (artificial periods) and to avoid endometrial hyperplasia.

UK/USA Drugs — Trade names		
	UK	**USA**
Androgens		
Testosterone enanthate	Primoteston Depot	Delatestryl
Testosterone cypionate		Depo-Testosterone Virilon IM
Testosterone (transdermal delivery)	Andropatch	Testoderm Androderm
Fluoxymesterone		Halotestin
Methyltestosterone		Testred Orethon Methyl
Nandrolone	Deca-Durabolin	Durabolin
Stanozol	Stromba	Winstrol
Oxymetholone		Anadrol 50
Anti-androgens and gonadotrophin release inhibitors		
Cyproterone acetate	Androcur	[Not approved for use in the USA]
Flutamide	Drogenil	Eulexin
Danazol	Danol	Danocrine
Oestrogens		
17β-Oestradiol	Zumenon	Emcyt Estrace
Piperazine oestrone sulphate [Estropipate]	Harmogen	Ortho-Est
Esterified oestrogens (mixture of sodium salts of sulphate esters of oestrogens, mainly oestrone)		Estratab Menest
Esterified oestrogens plus methyltestosterone		Estratest
Oestrogen antagonists		
Clomiphene	Clomid	Serophene
Tamoxifen	Tamofen, Noltam	Nolvadex
Progestogens		
Medroxyprogesterone	Provera Depo-Provera	Provera Depo-Provera
Norethindrone		Norlutin
Gonadotrophins (injectable)		
Urofollitrophin (FSH)	Metrodin	Metrodin
Human Chorionic Gonadotrophin (hCG)	Profasi Pregnyl	Profasi

References

Books

- **Braunstein GD.** (1994). Testes. In *Basic & Clinical Endocrinology*, edited by FS Greenspan, JD Baxter, 4th ed. Appleton & Lange, Connecticut, pp. 391–418

- **Ganong WF.** (1995). The gonads: development & function of the reproductive system. In *Review of Medical Physiology*, 17th ed. Appleton & Lange, Connecticut, pp. 379–417

- **Genuth SM.** (1993). The reproductive glands. In *Physiology*, edited by RM Berne, MN Levy, 3rd ed. Mosby-Year Book Inc., USA, pp. 980–1024

- **Goldfien A, Monroe SE.** (1994). Ovaries. In *Basic & Clinical Endocrinology*, edited by FS Greenspan, JD Baxter, 4th ed. Appleton & Lange, Connecticut, pp. 419–470

- **Goodman HM.** (1988). *Basic Medical Endocrinology*. Raven Press, New York, Chapters 11–12, pp. 253–302

- **Goldfein A** (1989). The gonadal hormones and inhibitors. In *Basic and Clinical Pharmacology*, edited by BG Katzung. Appleton & Lange, Connecticut, pp. 493–516

- **Griffin JE, Wilson JD.** (1987). Disorders of the testes/disorders of the ovary and female reproductive tract. In *Harrison's principles of internal medicine*, edited by E Braunwald, KJ Isselbacher *et al.*, 11th ed. McGraw-Hill, Inc., USA, Chapters 330–331, pp. 1807–1837

- **Griffin JE.** (1992). Male reproductive function. In *Textbook of Endocrine Physiology*, edited by JE Griffin, SR Ojeda, 2nd ed. Oxford University Press, New York, pp. 169–188

- **Harvey RA, Champe PC** *et al.* (1992). Steroid hormones. In *Lippincott's Illustrated Reviews: Pharmacology*. JB Lippincott Company, USA, pp. 243–252

- **Hedge GA, Colby HD, Goodman RL.** (1987). Endocrine systems. In *Clinical Endocrine Physiology*. WB Saunders Co., Philadelphia, Chapters 8–9, pp. 161–221

- **Junqueira LC, Carneiro J, Long JA.** (1986). The male/the female reproductive systems. In *Basic Histology*, 5th ed. Lange Medical Publications, Connecticut, Chapters 23–24, pp. 468–512

- **Laurence DR, Bennett PN.** (1992). Endocrinology IV: hypothalamic and pituitary hormones, sex hormones, contraception, uterus. In *Clinical Pharmacology*. Churchill Livingstone, pp. 591–614

- **Laycock J, Wise P** (1983). The gonads. In *Essential Endocrinology*, 2nd ed. Oxford University Press, Oxford, pp. 123–192

- **Martin J.** (1991). Contraception. In *Handbook of Pharmacy Health Education*. The Pharmaceutical Press, Chapter 4, pp. 73–97

- **Nachtigall RD.** (1992). Female reproductive disorders. In: *Handbook of Clinical Endocrinology*, edited by PA Fitzgerald, 2nd ed. Prentice-Hall, USA, pp. 402–462

- **Ojeda SR.** (1992). Female reproductive function. In *Textbook of Endocrine Physiology*, edited by JE Griffin, SR Ojeda, 2nd ed. Oxford University Press, New York, pp. 134–168

- **Rang HP, Dale MM, Ritter JM.** (1995). The reproductive system. In *Pharmacology*, 3rd ed. Churchill Livingstone, pp. 454–474

- **Sharlip ID.** (1992). Male reproductive disorders. In *Handbook of Clinical Endocrinology*, edited by PA Fitzgerald, 2nd ed. Prentice-Hall, USA, pp. 352–400

- **West JB.** (1991). The testis/the female reproductive system. In *Best and Taylor's Physiological Basis of Medical Practice*, 12th ed. Williams & Wilkins, Baltimore, Chapters 58–59, pp. 849–873

- **Williams CL. & Stancel GM.** (1996). Estrogens and progestins. In *Goodman & Gilman's The Pharmacological Basis of Therapeutics*, edited by JG Hardman, LE Limbird, A Goodman Gilman *et al.*, 9th ed. McGraw-Hill, USA, pp. 1411–1440

- **Wilson JD.** Androgens. In *Goodman & Gilman's The Pharmacological Basis of Therapeutics*, edited by JG Hardman, LE Limbird, A Goodman Gilman *et al.*, 9th ed. McGraw-Hill, USA, pp. 1441–1457

Journal Articles

- **Adashi EY.** (1994). Endocrinology of the ovary. *Hum Reprod*, 9, 815–827

- **Baird DT.** (1993). Antiestrogens. *Br Med Bull*, 49, 73–87

- **Craig Jordan V.** (1993). A current view of tamoxifen for the treatment and prevention of breast cancer. *Br J Pharmacol*, 110, 507–517

- **Gevers Leuven JA.** (1994). Sex steroids and lipoprotein metabolism. *Pharmac Ther*, 64, 99–126

- **Glasier A.** (1994). How and when to use postcoital contraception. *Prescriber*, 5(18), 59–63

- **Hampton N.** (1994). Hormonal contraceptives: their properties and uses. *Prescriber*, 5(12), 35–46

- **Huhtaniemi I.** (1994). Anabolic-androgenic steroids-a double edged sword? *Int J Androl*, 17, 57–62

- **Hillier SG.** (1994). Current concepts of the roles of follicle stimulating hormone and luteinizing hormone in folliculogenesis. *Hum Reprod*, 9, 188–191

- **Johnston A.** (1994). Management of the menopause with HRT. *Prescriber*, 5(19), 33–42

- **Knight PG.** (1996). Roles of inhibins, activins and follistatin in the female reproductive system. *Frontiers in Neuroendocrinol*, 17, 476–509

- **Kubba A, Guillebaud J.** (1993). Combined oral contraceptives: acceptability and effective use. *Br Med Bull*, 49, 140–157

- **Lee MM, Donahoe PK.** (1993). Mullerian inhibiting substance: A gonadal hormone with multiple functions. *Endocrine Rev*, 14, 152–164

- **Moore J.** (1997). Management and treatment options for endometriosis. *Prescriber*, 8(10), 73–76

- **Naftolin F** (1994). Brain aromatization of androgens. *J Reprod Med Obst Gynecol*, 39, 257–261

- **Prentice A.** (1994). Endometriosis: causes, diagnosis and treatment. *Prescriber*, 5(14), 27–34

- **Robustelli Della Cuna G, Pannuti F, Martoni A** *et al.* (1993). Aminoglutethimide in adrenal breast cancer: prospective randomized comparison of two dose levels. *Anticancer Res*, 13, 2367–2371

- **Session DR, Kelly AC, Jewelewicz, R.** (1993). Current concepts in estrogen replacement therapy in the menopause. *Fertil Steril*, 59, 277–284

- **Spitz IM, Bardin CW.** (1993). Clinical pharmacology of RU 486-an antiprogestin and antiglucocorticoid. *Contraception*, 48, 403–444

- **Thorogood M, Villard-Mackintosh L.** (1993). Combined oral contraceptives: risks and benefits. *Br Med Bull*, 49, 124–139

- **Smith C.** (1994). Norplant: a long-term hormonal contraceptive. *Prescriber*, 5(10), 19–23

- **Webb A.** (1997). A GP guide to non-oral methods of contraception. *Prescriber*, 8(4), 37–58

- **Woodruff TK, Mather JP.** (1995). Inhibin, activin and the female reproductive axis. *Annu Rev Physiol*, 57, 219–244

7 The Parathyroid Glands, Vitamin D and Hormonal Control of Calcium Metabolism

Calcium ions (Ca^{2+}) are necessary for bone and teeth formation, normal skeletal and smooth muscle function, cellular division adhesion and growth, blood coagulation, and for the normal activity of many intracellular enzymes. Calcium is also important for maintaining the activity of excitable tissue (acting as a membrane 'stabilizer') and is involved in neuromuscular transmission, cellular hormone release (*stimulus-secretion coupling*), and in the normal functioning of the heart.

The concentration of total extracellular calcium in the plasma is maintained within narrow limits (2.2–2.67 mmol/l; 8.4–10.7 mg/dl). By contrast, the *cytosolic* Ca^{2+} concentration is maintained at a very low level (10–100 nmol/l) by the active pumping of Ca^{2+} from the cytosol, and by uptake into mitochondria and the endoplasmic reticulum.

Plasma calcium exists in three forms:

1. *Free ionized* (50%). This is the metabolically and physiologically active form (ca. 1–1.4 mmol/l)
2. *Protein bound* (45%) — mainly to *albumin* and *globulins*
3. *Complexed with several anions* (5%) e.g. *bicarbonate, citrate, phosphate* and *sulphate*.

This distribution is influenced by the pH of the plasma, with a low plasma pH (*acidosis*) increasing free ionized calcium and *vice versa*.

Dietary calcium is mainly derived from white bread and dairy products such as milk, cheese and eggs. The calcium level of the body is influenced by dietary intake (ca. 1 g/day) and by the regulatory activity of three principal hormones, acting on bone, kidney and the intestinal tract (Figure 7.1):

1. **Parathyroid Hormone** — secreted by the *parathyroid glands*
2. **Calcitonin** — secreted by *thyroid parafollicular 'C' cells*
3. **1α,25-Dihydroxycholecalciferol** — a metabolite of Vitamin D.

Most (99%) of the body calcium is stored in bone. A fraction of this (readily exchangeable or labile pool) may be rapidly mobilized when necessary. Metabolism of **phosphate** (in the form of PO_4^{3-}, HPO_4^- and $H_2PO_4^-$), although not as finely controlled, is closely linked with that of calcium. Phosphate is necessary for the synthesis of many important molecules in the body e.g. nucleic acids (DNA, RNA), ATP, cAMP, membrane phospholipids (phosphatidylcholine) and is also an essential component of bone (as calcium phosphate and complex *hydroxyapatite salts*, containing calcium, phosphate and water). The normal plasma phosphate in adults is within the range 0.8–1.5 mmol/l (2.5–4.8 mg/dl).

The Parathyroid Glands
Structure and Histology

The **parathyroid glands**, consist of four ovoid-shaped bodies, each the size of a pea, embedded posteriorly in the four poles of the thyroid gland, within the thyroid capsule. Each gland is composed of densely packed epithelial cells of two distinct types, the *chief cells* and the *oxyphil cells*, surrounded by a thin layer of connective tissue. The *chief cells* are small and more numerous, with a clear cytoplasm containing small dense granules; these cells secrete **parathyroid hormone**, which regulates calcium and phosphate metabolism. The *oxyphil cells* are larger with a less granular cytoplasm, and have no known hormonal function.

Parathyroid Hormone

Parathyroid hormone (PTH) is an 84 amino acid linear peptide derived sequentially from larger precursor polypeptides, **prepro-PTH** and **pro-PTH** respectively. Following release, PTH is cleaved mainly by liver and kidney cells (plasma half-life ca. 2–5 min) to yield an active N-terminal portion containing the first 34 amino acids (residues 1–27 are essential), and an inactive C-terminal fragment; some cleavage also occurs within the parathyroid gland. The structure of human PTH is very similar to that of porcine or bovine PTH.

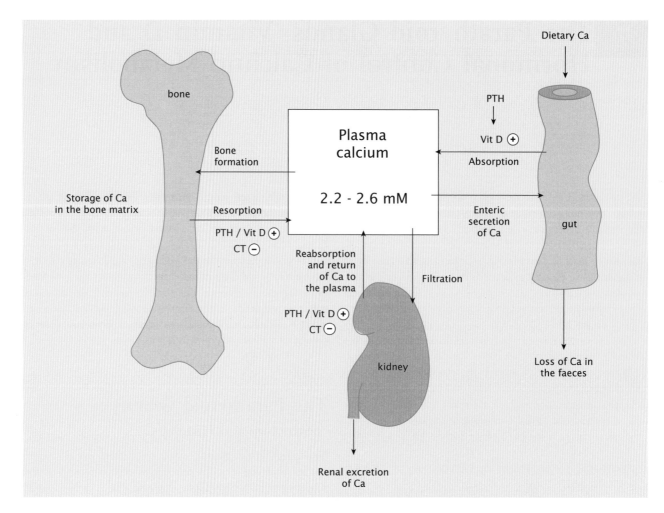

Figure 7.1. Calcium homeostasis. Major hormonal factors involved in the control of the plasma Ca^{2+} level, and their effects on the three principal target organs (bone, small intestine and kidney). Parathyroid hormone (PTH) and vitamin D (as $1,25$-$(OH)_2$ vitamin D_3) stimulate bone resorption and reabsorption of Ca^{2+} from the renal tubular fluid and small intestine, whereas calcitonin (CT) *inhibits* bone resorption and kidney reabsorption of Ca^{2+} with little effect on intestinal Ca^{2+} absorption. PTH stimulates gut absorption of Ca^{2+} *indirectly*, by stimulating the renal conversion of vitamin D to its active metabolite $1,25$-$(OH)_2$ vitamin D_3.

Control of Release

Unlike other endocrine hormones, PTH secretion is *not* controlled by the anterior pituitary gland: its secretion from parathyroid chief cells is determined by the circulating blood level of ionized Ca^{2+}. A *low* plasma Ca^{2+} concentration directly *stimulates* PTH release by the parathyroid glands, and a high level *suppresses* it (negative feedback). The latter effect is opposite to the more general effect of *intracellular* Ca^{2+} in *promoting* cellular hormone release, and is believed to involve a G-protein coupled cell-surface receptor for Ca^{2+} (*CaR1*). Plasma Mg^{2+} has a similar, though weaker effect than Ca^{2+} on PTH secretion; the physiological relevance of

this, however, is uncertain. Plasma phosphate levels have no *direct* effect on parathyroid PTH secretion. [The active vitamin D metabolite $1,25$-$(OH)_2D_3$ (see below) can, however, reduce PTH production by the parathyroid glands].

Principal Actions

The principal action of PTH is to *increase* plasma ionized calcium concentration: it is a *Ca^{2+}-raising factor*. This is achieved by influencing bone and renal tubular reabsorption of Ca^{2+}, and by increasing intestinal absorption. Plasma phosphate levels are *lowered* by PTH.

The main actions of PTH may be summarized as follows:

1. *In the kidney*, PTH causes a rapid increase in distal tubular reabsorption of Ca^{2+} (and Mg^{2+}) from the glomerular filtrate, and increases the excretion of phosphate in the urine (i.e. phosphate reabsorption via a *Na$^+$/phosphate-cotransport mechanism* in the proximal tubule is *inhibited*: the *phosphaturic* effect). Plasma Ca^{2+} concentration is therefore increased, while the plasma phosphate level falls. PTH also promotes the formation of the active vitamin D metabolite $1\alpha,25$-**dihydroxycholecalciferol** ($1,25$-$(OH)_2D_3$) within the kidney tubular cells, which in turn, facilitates the release of Ca^{2+} from bone and enhances the rate of absorption of Ca^{2+} from the small intestine and the kidney. Synthesis of $1,25$-$(OH)_2D_3$ is mediated through stimulation of the renal mitochondrial enzyme *25-hydroxyvitamin D-1α-hydroxylase*.

2. *On bone*, PTH has a dual action: it stimulates the rapid efflux of Ca^{2+} from the labile calcium pool across the *osteocyte-osteoblast bone membrane* (see below) into the extracellular fluid (facilitated by $1,25$-$(OH)_2D_3$); it also stimulates *osteoclast* bone cells (indirectly) to release calcium (and phosphate) by a slower process of *bone dissolution* or *resorption*, and increases the number of osteoclasts involved in this process. Eventually, *osteoblast* cells are also stimulated to synthesize new bone matrix.

3. *On the gastrointestinal tract*, PTH stimulates intestinal absorption of Ca^{2+} and phosphate indirectly. This effect (requiring 24 hours or longer) is mediated by the vitamin D metabolite $1,25$-$(OH)_2D_3$, and is therefore absent in vitamin D-deficient states. PTH stimulates the activity of the enzyme *1α-hydroxylase* involved in the production of $1,25$-$(OH)_2D_3$ in the kidney (see below).

Bone Cells Affected by Parathyroid Hormone

The two principal cell types in bone are *osteoblasts* and *osteoclasts*. **Osteoblasts** are specialized fibroblast-like cells (derived from marrow osteoprogenitor cells) responsible for new bone formation, by secreting type I collagen and glycoproteins into the extracellular space to form *osteoid*, which then calcifies to form an organic matrix containing initially, calcium phosphate (as $CaHPO_4.2H_2O$), and later, crystals of hydroxyapatite $[Ca_{10}(PO_4)_6(OH)_2]$ (mineralization). Osteoblasts that become entirely surrounded by mineralized bone are termed interior *osteocytes*; these cells maintain cytoplasmic contact with each other and with active osteoblasts via gap junctions (forming a 'bone membrane'). The enzyme *alkaline phosphatase* (believed to be important for normal bone mineralization), is present in osteoblast cells and appears in the plasma as a measure of osteoblastic activity.

Osteoclasts, on the other hand, are larger multinucleated cells (of haemopoietic origin) lining the bone-forming surface of bone tissue, that are capable of digesting previously formed bone matrix to release calcium and phosphate into the extracellular bone fluid (bone resorption); bone absorption occurs beneath the *ruffled border* area of the osteoclast, which releases hydrolytic enzymes (collagenase and proteinases) as well as protons. The slow continual (cyclic) process of resorption (lasting 2–4 weeks) is followed by new matrix deposition and mineralization (bone formation; lasting 3–7 months), so that total bone mass remains constant; this is known as *bone remodeling* (Figure 7.2) and is important for maintaining normal bone strength, repairing microfractures incurred during normal use, and for preserving calcium homeostasis. The sites on the bone surface at which remodeling occurs are termed *basic multicellular units (BMUs)*. It has been suggested that only osteoblast cells respond to PTH directly, and that the effects of PTH on osteoclast bone resorption are mediated indirectly through the release of *cytokines* (particularly *interleukins-1, and 6 [IL-1, IL-6]* and *granulocyte macrophage-colony stimulating factor [GM-CSF]*) which are responsible for activation and for differentiation of osteoclasts from precursor cells.

☞ Recently, a group of low molecular weight glycoproteins, **bone morphogenic proteins** (**BMPs 2-8**), belonging to the *transforming growth factor-β (TGF-β)* superfamily of regulatory proteins, have been isolated from bone matrix; [*BMP-7* (also known as *osteogenic protein-1: OP-1*) is actually synthesized within the kidney]. These molecules promote osteoblast and collagen cell (chondrocyte) differentiation from mesochymal stem cells, and may play an important role in cartilage and bone formation during embryonic development. Local implants containing *recombinant human BMP7 (hBMP7)* could prove useful in the future, for treating severe bone defects and for repairing tooth interiors.

Mechanism of Action

The effect of PTH on renal tubular and bone cell activity is believed to be mediated mainly via stimulation of specific plasma membrane receptors coupled through a G-protein to adenylate cyclase and a consequent rise in intracellular cAMP and cytosolic Ca^{2+}; [*an increased urinary excretion of cAMP occurs in direct response to PTH*]. Activation of other second messenger pathways (e.g. involving phosphoinositide metabolism, with production of *inositol trisphosphate [IP$_3$] and diacylglycerol [DAG]*) may also be involved in PTH actions.

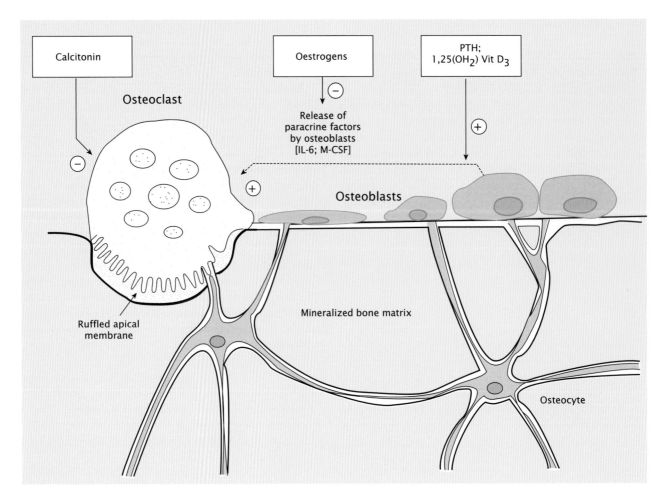

Figure 7.2. Bone remodeling by osteoblastic and osteoclastic cell activity. *Osteoclasts* are responsible for bone breakdown and de-mineralization (resorption) of mature bone, whereas *osteoblasts* form new bone and mineralize it. Parathyroid hormone (PTH) and 1,25-(OH)$_2$ vitamin D$_3$ stimulate osteoclastic bone resorption indirectly by facilitating release of osteoblastic cytokines (IL-6; GM-CSF), whereas calcitonin has a direct inhibitory effect on osteoclast activity. The inhibitory effects of oestrogens on resorption are thought to be mediated indirectly via inhibition of osteoblastic cytokine (IL-6) release.

☞ A **parathyroid hormone-related protein (PTHrP)**, secreted by a wide range of normal and malignant tissues, can also interact with the same membrane receptors as PTH in bone and kidney, and is believed to be responsible for the condition of *humoral hypercalcaemia of malignancy (HHM)* that can occur in ca. 10% of cancer patients (particularly with lung or breast carcinomas). PTHrP shares limited sequence homology with the 1–34 amino acid region of PTH. Recent studies also suggest that circulating PTHrP may have an important bone calcium mobilizing effect in the course of lactation, as well as other paracrine and/or autocrine effects independent of PTH receptor activation; [the PTHrP molecule can be post-translationally cleaved to yield a complex family of biologically active peptides].

Clinical Disorders

Hypersecretion (Hyperparathyroidism)

Primary hyperparathyroidism is a fairly prevalent, and slowly developing condition that is about 2–3 times more common in adult women than in men. The excess secretion of PTH causes *hyperclacaemia* and *phosphaturia* (excess loss of phosphate in the urine) resulting in a *low* plasma phosphate level (*hypophosphataemia*); a raised level of urinary cAMP may also be present. The disorder may be caused by a single chief cell tumour (adenoma) or enlargement of one or all four of the parathyroids (hyperplasia) or by a parathyroid carcinoma (rare). Hyperparathyroidism may also be associated with a more general inherited endocrine syndrome — *multiple endocrine neoplasia type 1 (MEN-1 disease)* also known as *multiple endocrine adenomatosis (MEA)*, involving many endocrine glands (e.g. pancreas, pituitary, adrenal or thyroid).

A *secondary* overactivity and hyperplasia of all four parathyroids (not associated with hypercalcaemia) can also develop as a compensatory response to longstanding *hypo*calcaemia due to intestinal calcium/vitamin D malabsorption (or deficiency) or chronic renal failure. PTH levels remain elevated until the cause of the hypocalcaemia can be corrected. *Mild hyperparathyroidism* may produce few clinical signs initially; however, *chronic PTH excess* may result in symptoms directly attributable to the elevated blood calcium level.

The main symptoms of hyperparathyroidism include:

1. *Tiredness*, general malaise, depression, weakness, lethargy, dizziness, excessive thirst, anorexia, nausea, vomiting and dehydration (due to excessive loss of urine), psychiatric disorders (depression, paranoia), cardiac arrhythmias (shortened QT interval on ECG recordings) and possible heart block. Anaemia and hypertension may be seen in some cases.
2. *Renal stones* (calculi) made from insoluble calcium phosphate (or oxalate), due to increased urinary excretion of Ca^{2+} and phosphate; this may cause renal colic and haematuria (appearance of blood in the urine), eventually leading to renal failure. *Gallstones* may also occur.
3. *Gastrointestinal complaints*: abdominal pain, constipation, dyspepsia, peptic and duodenal ulceration.
4. *Bone lesions* due to generalized loss (resorption) of calcium from bone. In severe cases, *osteitis fibrosa* (bone cysts) accompanied by bone pain and increased incidence of fractures can occur.
   Hyperparathyroidism has been described as a disease of '*bones, stones and abdominal groans*'.

Treatment. This is by careful surgical removal of the overactive parathyroid tissue (*subtotal parathyroidectomy*), although some tumours can be extremely difficult to locate (*ectopic* — at other sites). Parathyroid carcinomas can also be treated by local excision; however, postoperative persistence of hyperparathyroid symptoms or development of permanent *hypo*parathyroidism (with hypocalcaemia) are common. In rare instances, inadvertent damage to the recurrent laryngeal nerves may occur. Recurrence of the hyperparathyroid condition may require further surgery.

Severe hypercalcaemia (*hypercalcaemic crisis*) can be corrected by immediate administration of oral or intravenous rehydration fluids (normal saline solution) together with a loop diuretic (e.g. *frusemide*) to increase urinary Ca^{2+}

excretion; additional administration of **salmon calcitonin** (*Salcatonin; Calsynar*) (by subcutaneous or intramuscular injection) or slow intravenous infusion of **disodium pamidronate** (*Aredia*) (see below) to inhibit bone resorption may be necessary in some patients.

Future development of selective inhibitors of PTH action could provide a novel form of treatment for acute hyper-parathyroidism.

Hyposecretion (Hypoparathyroidism)

Lack of PTH causes *hypocalcaemia* and a high blood phosphate level (*hyperphosphataemia*) due to increased reabsorption of tubular phosphate. The most common cause is accidental damage of the parathyroids during thyroid surgery (*surgical hypoparathyroidism;* see Chapter 4). A rare form of primary (*idiopathic*) hypoparathyroidism can also result from autoimmune disease, usually co-existing with other organ-specific endocrine autoimmune disorders (e.g. adrenal insufficiency, hypothyroidism, type I diabetes); such individuals may possess specific serum antibodies directed against their parathyroid tissue.

☞ In the unusual hereditary condition of *pseudohyperparathyroidism*, parathyroid function is normal, but the primary target tissues (bone and kidney) are insensitive to the actions of PTH ('end-organ' resistance); this has been linked to a deficiency in the α-subunit structure of the stimulatory G_s-protein complex involved in PTH receptor transduction. Apart from a low plasma calcium level (ranging from mild to severe), affected patients show a characteristic rounded face, short stature, obesity, short fingers and may be mentally retarded.

A persistent low plasma calcium level can induce:

1. *Hyper-excitability of nerve and neuromuscular tissue*, characterized by a tingling sensation (*paraesthesia*: 'pins and needles') in the face or fingers, *muscle cramps* and *spasms* (particularly in the hands and feet) leading to hypocalcaemic tetany and even epileptic seizures/convulsions. A prolonged QT interval may be revealed on ECG recordings.
2. *Chvostek's sign* — a twitching of the facial muscles following light tapping over the facial nerve, and *Trousseau's sign* — a characteristic tetanic spasm of the wrist and fingers following over-inflation of a sphygmomanometer cuff placed over the upper arm for more than three minutes.
3. *Dental abnormalities, dry scaly skin and hair, brittle nails* and *cataracts* may also be present in more chronic persistent cases.

Treatment. Depending on the severity of the hypocalcaemia, this requires administration of vitamin D supplements in the form of **calciferol** tablets (*vitamin D₂*) or an oral solution of the vitamin D derivative **dihydrotacysterol** (*AT 10*) to enhance calcium absorption and utilization (see below); this must be coupled with frequent serum and urinary calcium measurements to ensure that *overtreatment* and consequent *hyper*calcaemia does not occur. Careful dose adjustment should then be made in order to maintain a normal blood calcium level. In acute cases of hypocalcaemic tetany, a more rapid elevation in blood calcium may be achieved by means of an intravenous infusion of *10% calcium gluconate solution* given over 10 mins or longer as needed to counteract symptoms. PTH itself is not available for replacement therapy.

Calcitonin

Calcitonin (CT) is a 32 amino acid single-chain peptide hormone secreted by the parafollicular 'C' cells of the thyroid gland (see Chapter 4). It is derived from larger precursor peptides **pre-procalcitonin** and **procalcitonin** respectively, and stored in secretory vesicles within the parafollicular cells from which it is released by exocytosis [some procalcitonin and a dimeric form of calcitonin are also released, both being inactive]. The entire amino acid sequence of the molecule is required for significant biological activity, although interestingly, the structures of human and animal (porcine, bovine, ovine) calcitonins vary considerably (by up to 19 amino acids). The fish and avian calcitonin molecules show the highest degree of activity compared with other calcitonins.

Control of Release

The main factor involved in regulating calcitonin release from 'C' cells is the free ionized Ca^{2+} concentration in the blood. A *rise* in plasma Ca^{2+} *stimulates* calcitonin release, and *vice versa* [note the opposite effect of Ca^{2+} on PTH secretion]. Release of calcitonin is also promoted by the gastrointestinal hormone **gastrin**, which could be an important feedback mechanism guarding against the development of hypercalcaemia following a meal. The plasma half-life of calcitonin is relatively short (2–15 min) due to rapid degradation of the peptide in the plasma and kidney.

Principal Actions

Unlike PTH, calcitonin is a Ca^{2+}-lowering factor; it *decreases* plasma calcium (and phosphate) levels principally by:

1. *Decreasing* the efflux of Ca^{2+} across the osteocyte-osteoblast bone membrane and also by inhibiting bone resorption through a direct suppression of osteoclast bone cell activity and a decreased formation of new osteoclasts from bone marrow precursors. The effects of calcitonin are greater when the rate of bone resorption is high.

2. *Inhibiting* renal tubular reabsorption of calcium and phosphate (from ascending loop of Henle and distal tubules). Calcitonin has no significant effect on intestinal Ca^{2+} fluxes.

Although these effects are generally *opposite* to those of PTH (physiological antagonism), calcitonin is not considered to be as important as PTH and vitamin D in the normal regulation of calcium or skeletal homeostasis in humans. Calcitonin affects target tissues (e.g. osteoclast cells) by interacting with specific surface membrane receptors linked to the production of intracellular cAMP. The areas of the kidney tubule that respond to calcitonin are different from those responding to PTH.

Clinical Disorders

Clinical disorders involving calcitonin under or over secretion are very rare. Excessive secretion of calcitonin (together with some dimeric and polymeric molecular forms) can however, be produced by certain *medullary thyroid carcinomas* (derived from parafollicular 'C' cells) or by ectopic tumours (e.g. in the lung or breast). In such cases, there is no significant imbalance in plasma calcium and phosphate levels, but the excess calcitonin can be useful as a tumour marker. Similarly, removal of the thyroid gland in thyrotoxicosis, does not result in overt hypercalcaemia.

Therapeutic Uses

The two main therapeutic uses of calcitonin are in the treatment of severe *Paget's disease of bone* and the management of *severe hypercalcaemic states*:

1. *Paget's disease* is a common chronic disorder of unknown cause (possibly viral) that affects ca. 0.5% of the population (particularly men) over the age of 40. It is characterized by an abnormally high level of bone turnover due to excessive osteoclastic bone resorption, followed by increased activity of osteoblasts, attempting to repair the bone damage. The affected bones (usually the skull, spine, pelvis and long bones) ultimately become deformed and show an abnormal density under X-ray. Despite the increased bone turnover, the condition is initially largely asymptomatic; plasma Ca^{2+} and phosphate levels are normal, although an elevated level of *alkaline phosphatase* (reflecting osteoblastic cell activity and bone turnover) may be present.

Clinical features include: *joint and bone pain, fractures, bone deformities* — particularly affecting the legs ('bowed' tibia), and *skull enlargement*, leading to auditory and optic nerve compression (*deafness/blindness*).

Porcine calcitonin (from pork parathyroids: *Calcitare*) or **salcatonin** (synthetic salmon calcitonin: *Miacalcic; Calsynar;* expensive!) may be given daily by subcutaneous or intramuscular injection over 3–6 months to reduce bone resorption, improve bone abnormalities and relieve the bone pain and neurological complications associated with the disease; *nausea* and *facial flushing* can occur as *side effects*. Prolonged use may also result in neutralizing antibodies against calcitonin being formed (salcatonin is less immunogenic).

☞ Other drugs (**bisphosphonates**; analogues of pyrophosphate, a natural inhibitor of bone mineralization) are also available for treatment of Paget's disease of bone; these compounds reduce osteoclastic bone resorption by a dual mechanism: they are adsorbed strongly onto bone hydroxyapatite crystals (especially at bone remodeling sites) and slow their rate of formation and dissolution, and they also inhibit osteoclast cell activity indirectly, by decreasing the production of osteoclast-stimulating factors by osteoblasts. **Disodium etidronate** (*Didronel*) tablets may be given daily for 3–6 months (avoiding food two hr before or after taking doses). *Unwanted effects* are few and include: *nausea, diarrhoea* and a temporary *metallic/altered taste sensation.*

Oral **disodium etidronate** (*Didronel PMO*), alternating with a calcium carbonate supplement, taken on an intermittent cyclical basis (two weeks etidronate. 76 days calcium every three months, for up to 3 years) or subcutaneous **salcatonin** [expensive!] (daily, together with dietary calcium and vitamin D supplements for 2–3 years) have been found effective in increasing bone mineral content and preventing excessive bone loss in established *postmenopausal vertebral osteoporosis:* (see below) [useful for patients that are unable or unwilling to take HRT; Chapter 6]. A recently introduced (more potent) oral bisphosphonate **sodium alendronate** (*Fosamax*) can be administered continuously (with calcium supplementation) for this purpose, with no restriction on the duration of treatment. Intranasal preparations of **salcatonin** are available in the USA (*Miacalcin*) and in some European countries, but not currently in the UK.

2. *Hypercalcaemic states.* Porcine calcitonin or salcatonin (subcutaneous or intramuscular) can be used to produce a rapid (within 24 hr) reduction in the plasma Ca^{2+} concentration in some patients with hypercalcaemia (particularly when induced by malignant disease: see above). In severe cases, a slow intravenous infusion of salcatonin may be given. Long-term use of calcitonin or salcatonin over several months can however, lead to clinical resistance due to a down-regulation of calcitonin receptors on target tissues and (in the case of the former), the development of neutralizing plasma antibodies.

Slow intravenous infusion of bisphosphonate drugs e.g. **disodium pamidronate** (*Aredia*) or **sodium clodronate** (*Loron; Bonefos*) are also now widely used in the control of tumour-induced hypercalcaemia of malignancy.

Vitamin D

This term describes a group of essential fat soluble *sterols* with a steroid-like structure, which can influence calcium and phosphate metabolism. Although traditionally regarded as a vitamin (essential food nutrient), it is more correctly classified as a hormone, since it can be produced endogenously in small amounts within one organ and travels via the blood to affect the activity of cells at distant sites. Vitamin D ingested from dietary sources or synthesized in the skin after sunlight exposure is biologically inert, and must undergo successive transformation in the liver and kidneys to produce an active form **1α,25-dihydroxycholecalciferol** ($1,25\text{-}(OH)_2D_3$) before being released into the bloodstream to affect a wide variety of target tissues — principally the small intestine, bone and kidney. Other target tissues include the brain, bone marrow, lymphocytes, spinal cord, endocrine pancreas and other endocrine cells, skin keratinocytes, breast tissue, and the male and female reproductive organs; however, the physiological relevance of vitamin D action at many of these sites is not yet entirely clear.

☞ $1,25\text{-}(OH)_2D_3$ is known to be a potent stimulator of cell differentiation and an inhibitor of proliferation, and may therefore be important in the growth and development of certain tissues, particularly immune cells and keratinocytes. In addition there is increasing evidence favouring a role for vitamin D in the modulation of seasonal and daily (light-driven) biorhythms (unrelated to its effects on calcium homeostasis) through its effects on the brain and endocrine tissues.

Vitamin D is found mainly in two forms:

1. **Vitamin D_2** (*calciferol; ergocalciferol*), a plant-derived vitamin, produced by solar ultraviolet light irradiation of a plant sterol (ergosterol) and contained in most clinically available preparations.

2. **Vitamin D_3** (*cholecalciferol*), the natural animal vitamin D, synthesized within the skin of man and higher mammals from an inactive precursor *7-dehydrocholesterol*

(provitamin D_3) by the ultraviolet effect of sunlight (300–320 nm wavelength). To become active, it is first hydroxylated in the liver to *25-hydroxy-cholecalciferol* (25-$(OH)D_3$) and then to the active form **1α,25-dihydroxycholecalciferol** (1,25-$(OH)_2D_3$; *calcitriol*) in the proximal convoluted tubules of the kidneys, under the influence of **parathyroid hormone**; [some production of 1,25-$(OH)_2D_3$ from 25-$(OH)D_3$ also takes place in the skin]. 1,25-$(OH)_2D_3$ is also often referred to as **soltriol** or the *'heliogenic' steroid hormone*. 1,25-$(OH)_2D_3$ can regulate its own production by inhibiting the renal *25-hydroxyvitamin D-1α-hydroxylase* enzyme activity and also by inducing kidney *24-hydroxylase* enzyme activity to yield the weakly active metabolite *24,25-$(OH)_2D_3$* (Figure 7.3). Phosphate depletion also stimulates 1-α-hydroxylase activity, leading to an increased formation of 1,25-$(OH)_2D_3$.

1,25-$(OH)_2D_3$ is transported in the blood largely bound to a specific vitamin D-binding α-globulin, *transcalciferin* (which can also bind vitamin D_3 and 25-$(OH)D_3$), secreted mainly by the liver; as with other steroidal hormones (see Chapters 3 and 6), only the free unbound 1,25-$(OH)_2D_3$ is biologically active (plasma half-life ca. 3–6 h). The daily requirement of vitamin D to maintain calcium homeostasis in adults is very small (ca. 10 μg/day).

☞ Vitamin D_2 (*calciferol*) differs from vitamin D_3 in having an additional double bond between side chain positions C_{22-23} and a methyl group attached at C_{24} (Figure 7.3). In humans, following ingestion and absorption by the small intestine (incorporated into *chylomicrons*), it is metabolised via similar pathways to yield *1α,25-dihydroxycalciferol* (1,25-$(OH)_2D_2$), which is equivalent in biological activity to 1,25-$(OH)_2D_3$.

Principal Actions

1,25-$(OH)_2D_3$ promotes the active absorption of calcium from the upper small intestine (main action) and from bone and kidney (weak action), with a secondary increase in phosphate absorption. Like the steroid hormones (see Chapters 3 and 6), the action of 1,25-$(OH)_2D_3$ on its target tissues is mediated by a specific cytosolic vitamin D receptor protein (VDR) which then interacts with DNA within the cell nucleus to activate specific genes; in the intestine and kidney, this results in the enhanced synthesis of cytosolic *calcium binding proteins [CaBP(9K) and CaBP(28K)* also termed *calbindins]* as well a transporter pump protein (*Ca-Mg-ATPase*) involved in calcium absorption. The VDR is considered to be a 'primitive' form of the thyroid hormone receptor protein (TR), possibly having evolved from the same primordial gene. Consequently, the effect of 1,25-

$(OH)_2D_3$ may show a lag period of 1–3 days before the plasma calcium level rises: [genetic susceptibility of individuals to osteoporosis (see below) may be linked to molecular variations in the structure of the VDR].

1,25-$(OH)_2D_3$ may also exert a more rapid, directly-mediated stimulation of duodenal Ca^{2+} transport by a non-genomic mechanism (*transcaltachia*), most likely involving a separate receptor system with a different conformational requirement for the hormone ligand.

The action of 1,25-$(OH)_2D_3$ on osteoclast bone resorption may be *indirectly* mediated by release of paracrine factors from stimulated osteoblast cells; (only osteoblasts possess intracellular VDRs). 1,25-$(OH)_2D_3$ also induces an increase in the synthesis and release of the bone-specific protein *osteocalcin* by osteoblasts, which is deposited in the matrix and could be involved in osteoclast recruitment or activation. Plasma osteocalcin levels (together with alkaline phosphatase) are useful clinical metabolic markers of bone osteoblastic activity.

Clinical Disorders

DEFICIENCY OF VITAMIN D

This causes *rickets* in young children and *osteomalacia* (soft bones) in adults (particularly heavily-veiled female immigrants living in the UK, and in housebound elderly). Both conditions still occur quite commonly in tropical and subtropical countries, and are characterized by an inadequate calcification of the bone matrix and a softening of the skeleton.

In children the growing ends of bone are swollen, and the bone becomes bent and deformed, giving a characteristic 'bowed legs' appearance.

In adults the main feature is bone pain, partial bone fractures and muscle weakness (which may lead to falls).

☞ A natural decrease in the ability of the skin to synthesize vitamin D_3 occurs with increasing age.

Vitamin D deficiency may be due to a metabolic abnormality (e.g. inherited *absence or reduced renal 1α-hydroxylase activity (vitamin D-dependent rickets type 1 [VDDR 1])*, *intestinal fat malabsorption*, *chronic liver disease*, *insufficient exposure to sunlight* or simple *dietary lack*; [the main sources of vitamin D include fish, liver, eggs, cod liver oil and fortified milk, cereals and margarine].

Treatment of simple dietary deficiency involves giving small oral doses of vitamin D (up to 10 μg daily; 400 units[*]) to enhance calcium absorption, together with a calcium supplement if necessary.

[*][1 unit ≡ 25 ng of vitamin D_2 or D_3.]

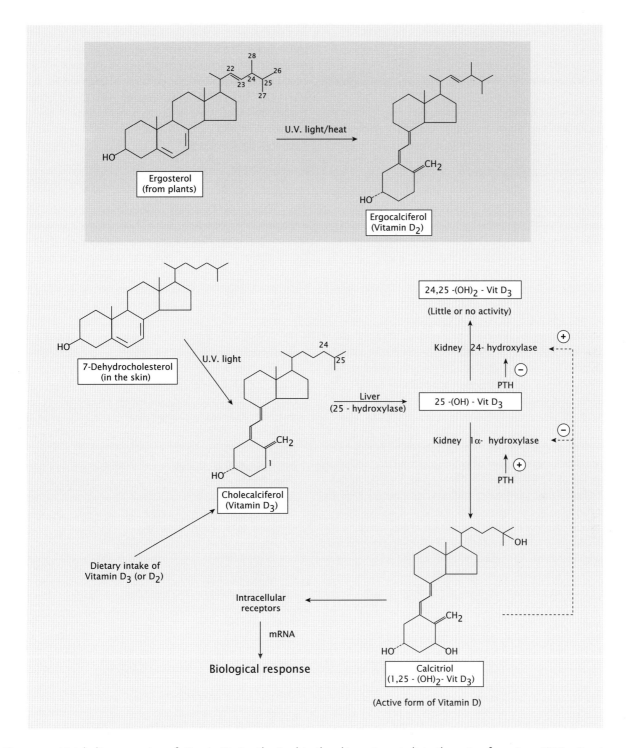

Figure 7.3. Metabolic conversion of vitamin D₃ (synthesized in the skin or ingested) to the active form (1,25-(OH)₂ vitamin D₃) via liver 25-hydroxylase and kidney 1α-hydroxylase enzyme activity respectively. Parathyroid hormone (PTH) stimulates 1α-hydroxylase activity but inhibits 24-hydroxylase activity in the kidney. 1,25-(OH)₂ vitamin D₃ can regulate its own production by stimulating 24-hydroxylase activity to produce the inactive metabolite 24,25-(OH)₂ vitamin D₃, and also by *inhibiting* 1α-hydroxylase activity (negative feedback).

The transformation of the plant precursor steroid ergosterol to vitamin D₂ (ergocalciferol) by the action of UV light and heat is also shown above. Ergocalciferol is converted (after ingestion in humans) to its corresponding active form 1,25-(OH)₂D₂ by the liver and kidney.

Currently available vitamin D supplement preparations include:

1. **Chocovite tablets** (*Ca gluconate with 1.25 μg vitamin D$_2$*)

2. **Calcichew D3 tablets** (*Ca carbonate with 5 μg vitamin D$_3$*) or **Calcium and ergocalciferol (vitamin D$_2$) tablets** (*Ca lactate and phosphate with 10 μg vitamin D$_2$*);

☞ Chronic administration of certain anticonvulsant drugs (e.g. **phenytoin** or **phenobarbitone**) that cause induction of hepatic microsomal enzymes, can increase the rate of clearance of vitamin D metabolites from the body and therefore induce symptoms of vitamin D deficiency; oral vitamin D supplements may be preventative in such cases.
In cases of intestinal malabsorption or hepatic disease, higher vitamin D doses (up to 1 mg daily) may be necessary in the form of higher strength preparations:

3. **Calciferol** (*ergocalciferol, vitamin D$_2$*) or **cholecalciferol** (*vitamin D$_3$*) (in 250 μg tablets, or by intramuscular injection in vegetable oil); [1.25 mg tablets are also available for treatment of *hypoparathyroidism* which may require doses up to 2.5 mg daily].

Treatment of severe rickets or osteomalacia may require a large intramuscular dose of vitamin D initially, followed by regular oral supplements. Patients with renal impairment who cannot adequately hydroxylate vitamin D to its active form, may be treated with the newer active derivatives **alfacalcidiol** (*1α-hydroxycholecalciferol: One-Alpha; AlfaD*) or **calcitriol** (*1α,25-dihydroxycholecalciferol: Calcijex; Rocaltrol*) given in the form of capsules, oral solution or by slow intravenous injection; these analogues have a more rapid onset and a shorter duration of action than vitamin D$_2$ or D$_3$. Calcitriol can also be used for treating patients with the metabolic VDDR 1 abnormality.

All patients taking high doses of vitamin D preparations require regular monitoring of their plasma and urinary Ca^{2+} concentration (particularly in early stages of treatment) to check for development of hypercalcaemia and possible vitamin D toxicity.

☞ Vitamin D supplements should be avoided by women during lactation, since excess vitamin D secreted into breast milk could induce hypercalcaemia in infants.

Vitamin D-Dependent Rickets Type 2 [VDDR 2]

This disease (also known as vitamin D-resistant rickets) is a relatively common hereditary condition caused by a de-

fect in the gene encoding the 1,25-(OH)$_2$D$_3$ receptor; such individuals develop a nutritional-type rickets but show a resistance to physiological doses of vitamin D and its metabolites, despite having high plasma levels of 1,25-(OH)$_2$D$_3$. Patients with this disorder will therefore require higher doses of vitamin D or vitamin D metabolites for treatment; severe *alopecia* (hair-loss) of uncertain cause, may also be present.

Vitamin D Excess (Hypervitaminosis D)

Hypervitaminosis D usually results from overtreatment with a vitamin D preparation. Initial hypercalcaemic symptoms include tiredness, loss of appetite and nausea. It may also occur spontaneously (with resultant hypercalcaemia) in some patients with *sarcoidosis*, where an enhanced synthesis of vitamin D$_3$ (and a consequent increase in production of 1,25-(OH)$_2$D$_3$) occurs in the skin after sun exposure.

☞ *Sarcoidosis* is a chronic (usually benign) systemic disease of unknown cause, in which nodules of inflamed tissue (*granulomas*) infiltrate the skin and other body organs e.g. lungs, lymph nodes, liver, and the spleen. These bodies consist of compact accumulations of epithelioid cells, monocytes and macrophages, that may be induced by toxic irritants or other unknown antigens. The condition can appear as a localized inflammation of the skin on the shins (*erythema nodosum*), but can also affect other body areas (face, hands, eyes). Skin sarcoidosis is characterized by a hypersensitivity to vitamin D and development of hypercalcaemic symptoms in some patients after prolonged exposure to sunlight or excessive ingestion of vitamin D-containing products. The increased metabolism of vitamin D is thought to occur within the sarcoid macrophages and lymphoid cells associated with the granulomatous follicles. The condition responds well to systemic or local corticosteroid therapy and may resolve spontaneously after a few years.

Keratinocyte Differentiation

In addition to their important role in synthesizing vitamin D$_3$, skin keratinocytes are also capable of producing 1,25-(OH)$_2$D$_3$ from circulating 25-(OH)D$_3$, which in turn exerts a localized function (together with Ca^{2+}) to regulate keratinocyte differentiation. The synthetic vitamin D analogues **calcipotriol** and **tacalcitol** stimulate the differentiation and inhibit the proliferation of keratinocytes, and have proved useful (as an alternative to corticosteroid therapy) in the topical treatment of psoriasis (*Dovonex* cream; *Curatoderm* ointment). Regular monitoring of the plasma calcium level is not considered necessary during usage since calcipotriol possesses only weak 'calcaemic' activity.

The arrival of newer systemically active 'non-calcaemic' vitamin D analogues in the future, could provide a useful and novel class of antitumour drugs for the treatment of cancer.

Other Hormones Affecting Calcium Homeostasis

Gonadal Steroids

Oestrogens have a well recognized role in maintaining the bone mass in women, by preventing bone resorption. After the menopause when oestrogen levels decrease, the imbalance between bone resorption and bone formation may lead to *osteoporosis* (decalcification of bone and reduction in bone density) which in some women could lead to bone fragility and potentially fatal hip and vertebral compression fractures [in men, testosterone has a similar function in protecting against the development of osteoporosis]. Oestrogen deficiency also increases the sensitivity of the bone to PTH, by an unknown mechanism. Oestrogens have an inhibitory effect on osteoclast cell activity (and hence bone resorption), however oestrogen receptors (that also bind androgens) are present predominantly in osteoblast cells; their main protective effects may therefore be mediated indirectly, by inhibiting the release of specific osteoclast-activating/differentiating factors from osteoblasts (e.g. *IL-6* and *granulocyte-macrophage-colony stimulating factor [GM-CSF]*) and also from peripheral blood monocytes (*interleukin-1 [IL-1], tumour necrosis factor-α [TNF-α] and GM-CSF*) [a direct inhibitory action of oestrogens on osteoclast function may also occur]. Osteoblasts also respond to oestrogen by increasing their production of the paracrine factor *transforming growth factor beta (TGF-β)* which has an inhibitory effect on osteoclastic activity. In addition, progestogens can stimulate new bone formation by binding to osteoclast cells (facilitated by oestrogens). It has been suggested that the main protective effects of androgens on bone turnover in men could involve an intermediate local aromatization into oestrogens via skeletal aromatases.

Glucocorticoids

Glucocorticoids administered in high (pharmacologic) doses or chronically present in excess in patients with Cushing's syndrome (see Chapter 3) are known to affect bone metabolism and calcium turnover, leading ultimately to a characteristic *'glucocorticoid-induced osteoporosis'*. The precise mechanisms responsible for this bone loss, however, are incompletely understood. High concentrations of glucocorticoids inhibit osteoblastic bone formation and stimulate PTH-mediated bone resorption by osteoclasts resulting in an 'uncoupling' of the bone remodeling cycle. High affinity glucocorticoid receptors have been demonstrated in osteoblasts, but not osteoclast cells, indicating that the effects of glucocorticoids on bone resorption are indirect. The vitamin D-induced production of the marker protein *osteocalcin* by osteoblasts is also suppressed via an action at the $1,25\text{-}(OH)_2D_3$ receptor level. Other factors contributing to the glucocorticoid effect include a decrease in Ca^{2+} absorption from the gut (by a vitamin D-independent mechanism) and an increase in urinary excretion of Ca^{2+} (reduction in renal Ca^{2+} reabsorption), leading to a fall in plasma calcium level.

Growth Hormone

Growth hormone (GH) is essential for promoting longitudinal bone growth of the skeleton (see Chapter 2). Recent studies of the effects of prolonged treatment of elderly individuals with *biosynthetic human growth hormone (hGH)* (produced using recombinant DNA technology) indicate that hGH can effectively inhibit age-related loss of bone mineral. The safety and efficacy of chronically-administrated hGH in such cases however, remains to be fully evaluated, and this form of therapy at current prices of the hormone, would be very expensive in the long run. Treatment with hGH may also have other important benefits in the elderly, including improved muscle strength and reduction in adiposity.

Osteoporosis

Osteoporosis refers to a group of metabolic bone disorders characterized by a decreased bone mass (*osteopenia*). The bone (particularly trabecular) becomes abnormally thin and porous, due to an uncompensated loss of bone mineral and matrix. Along with a progressive decrease in bone mass, there is a micro-architectural deterioration of osteoporotic bone tissue, contributing further to the ease with which fractures occur. The prevalence of osteoporosis increases with age in both sexes, although women are more prone to develop the condition after the menopause. Increasingly, men are also being diagnosed with the condition, although a generally lower incidence in males would be expected, partly due to their larger initial bone mass, and partly because of the protective anabolic effects of secreted androgens.

Primary osteoporosis may be classified into two main clinical types: *postmenopausal (oestrogen-deficiency; type I)* and *age-related (senile; type II)*. The former is seen in women between the ages of 55–75 years, and is attributed to the lack of ovarian oestrogens, whereas the latter is commonly found in both men and women between 70–75 years, and attributed to a progressive inefficiency of the bone remodeling process and decrease in renal 1,25-(OH)$_2$D$_3$ formation/gastrointestinal Ca^{2+} absorption with age.

The major increase in bone mass occurs during adolescence, attaining a peak in early adulthood (ca. 30 years of age), and thereafter declines steadily during adult life, due to a cumulative remodeling-induced deficit. Early bone acquisition is dependent upon adequate dietary intake of calcium, circulating levels of oestrogens/androgens and physical activity, as well as other genetically programmed factors. In the elderly, bone density will thus be determined by their peak bone mass attained in early adulthood and the subsequent bone loss; after the age of 55–60 years, both sexes lose bone at a rate of ca. 1% per year. Bone loss can also be increased by certain endocrine disorders (see below), long-term administration of glucocorticoids, or prolonged immobilization. Following menopause, the rate of bone loss in women is significantly accelerated due to loss of oestrogen production (about 15% of bone is lost within five to ten years). Men avoid this rapid menopausal bone loss seen in women, and consequently have a lower susceptibility to bone fractures.

In osteoporosis, as in hypertension, there is often a long latent period before clinical symptoms and signs become evident, therefore patients may show no initial symptoms. However, when they do occur, **the major symptoms are:**

1. *Bone pain* due to a fracture (occurring spontaneously or following minimal trauma), or severe back pain due to vertebral collapse.

2. *Loss of height* and *dorsal kyphosis* (curvature of the spine; *dowager's hump*). These are classic signs of more well-established osteoporosis.

3. *Fractures.* Since osteoporosis increases the fragility of the entire skeleton, fractures may occur anywhere, but typical sites include the hip (most dangerous), vertebrae, ribs, distal radius (*Colles' fracture*), humerus and proximal femur. A greater tendency to fall with increasing age is a further important factor governing the incidence of fractures.

Such fractures create a major public health and disability problem for elderly men and women in the western world, leading to a considerable number of premature deaths. The annual fracture burden (ca. 150,000 cases/year in the UK) imposed on the health services in the UK as the result of osteoporotic (mostly hip) fractures has been estimated at £742 million.

Risk Factors

Several risk factors are recognized: female gender; a tall slender body build (<58 kg); Caucasian racial origin; blonde hair colour; family history of hip; wrist or spine fracture; cigarette smoking; alcoholism (which reduces osteoblastic activity); excessive caffeine intake; lack of weight-bearing exercise; prolonged immobility; deficiency of gonadal hormones; endocrine abnormalities such as Cushing's syndrome, hyperparathyroidism, hyperthyroidism and hyperprolactinaemia with hypogonadism. Women athletes and ballet dancers suffering from secondary amenorrhoea may also show an accelerated bone loss (also found in women with chronic anorexia nervosa).

Osteoporosis is also seen in dietary vitamin C or D deficiency (or abnormalities in the vitamin D receptor gene), renal tubular acidosis, chronic renal, liver or inflammatory bowel disease, rheumatoid arthritis, and in certain genetic disorders such as *osteogenesis imperfecta* (brittle bone syndrome) and *homocystinuria* (an inborn error of amino acid metabolism).

Bone Density Measurements

Non-invasive, quantitative measures of bone mass are a valuable indicator of bone strength and fracture risk in osteoporotic patients, and are also useful in the evaluation of therapeutic interventions. Bone mineral density (BMD) can now be measured precisely at selected skeletal sites prone to osteoporotic fractures, e.g. the lumbar spine (L2–L4) or femoral neck, using low irradiation *dual-energy X-ray absorptiometry (DXA)*. Alternative methods currently in use include *single or dual-photon absorptiometry (SPA, DPA)* or *quantitative computerized tomography (QCT)* [regular calibration of instruments is essential]. In general, the risk of bone fracture increases as BMD decreases: osteoporosis is considered to be present when BMD is more than 2.5 standard deviations below the expected mean for young (20–40 year old) healthy adults of the same gender [a BMD value ≤1 SD below the young adult mean is regarded as normal].

Prevention and Treatment

Treatment of osteoporosis emphasizes prevention as the most effective therapy, since lost bone mass in this disorder is difficult to replace. No drug yet exists that can reverse the effects of osteoporosis. Adequate dietary intake of calcium or oral calcium supplementation in the form of tablets (or effervescent formulations) containing Ca gluconate, lactate or carbonate salts (*Calcit; Calcichew; Sandocal*) is thus very crucial in the perimenopausal period; women in their reproductive years should consume about 1 g of calcium per day, whereas in pregnant or lactating women, or after the postmenopause, the requirement is about 1.5 g daily. Taking regular moderate physical exercise (especially walking) and avoiding cigarette smoking, excess alcohol consumption and drugs like steroids, especially during adolescence and young adulthood, should also help in maintaining bone mass.

In postmenopausal women, oestrogen replacement as part of HRT (see Chapter 6) is the most effective method of decreasing the rapid bone loss and reducing fracture rate in both the spine and the hip. To be fully effective, HRT should preferably be started within the first 5 years following menopause and continued for at least 5–10 years. Although some benefit is seen when the treatment is begun later, it is significantly less pronounced. In women with an intact uterus, combined oestrogen/progestogen HRT is necessary to reduce the risk of developing endometrial cancer (see Table 6.3). The usefulness of long-term androgen replacement therapy (e.g. using transdermal testosterone patches: *Andropatch; [Testoderm; Androderm: USA]*) in hypogonadal men with osteoporosis remains unclear.

Other main pharmacologic approaches include antiresorptive agents such as **salcatonin** (given by daily subcutaneous or intramuscular injection or by intranasal spray [*Miacalcin: USA*] together with oral calcium and vitamin D supplements) or oral bisphosphonates taken on an intermittent cyclical basis (**disodium etidronate**; *Didronel PMO*) or administered continuously (**sodium alendronate**; *Fosamax*) (both with calcium supplementation). The increase in spinal BMD achieved with the bisphosphonates is associated with an ca. 50% decrease in vertebral fracture rate, comparable to that seen with HRT. For elderly patients over 75 years of age, the use of antiresorptive agents is not considered to be beneficial; modest amounts of vitamin D (20 µg daily) taken together with a calcium supplement may then be the most effective method for reducing fracture risk among such people.

The possible use of an oral slow-release form of **sodium fluoride** (given with calcium) to stimulate bone formation in post-menopausal osteoporosis and decrease vertebral fracture rate is controversial. Another novel form of 'anabolic' therapy currently being evaluated, involves the administration of daily subcutaneous injections of the 1–34 amino acid fragment of *human parathyroid hormone [hPTH (1–34); teriparatide]* which, in low doses, stimulates osteoblastic bone formation without affecting blood Ca^{2+} levels. Future development of intranasally or oral formulations of this (or related PTH fragments) could thus provide an exciting new therapeutic approach for the treatment of osteoporosis.

Raloxifene hydrochloride is a non-steroidal tissue-specific oestrogen receptor ligand (or *selective oestrogen receptor modulator, SERM*) that is currently being evaluated as an effective alternative to HRT in the treatment of osteoporosis in post-menopausal women, but may also be useful in preventing the development of breast and endometrial cancers. This novel benzothiopene compound acts as a selective oestrogen agonist on bone, but unlike oestradiol, is an oestrogen antagonist on other tissue; it is therefore free of endometrial hyperplastic effects, and should not increase the risk of endometrial cancer. ∎

Review Questions

Question 1: Explain the physiological importance of Ca^{2+} in the body.

Question 2: State the normal concentration of total calcium in the plasma and name the three hormones involved in calcium regulation.

Question 3: List the three forms in which calcium exists in the plasma.

Question 4: State the major forms of inorganic phosphate in the body.

Question 5: Describe the location, and structure of the parathyroid glands; name their principal hormone secretion, and state its effect on the plasma Ca^{2+} level.

Question 6: Describe the mechanisms controlling parathyroid hormone (PTH) release.

Question 7: Describe the main actions of PTH on:
  a) the kidney,
  b) bone resorption,
  c) the gastrointestinal tract.

Question 8: State the two principal types of bone cell and outline their function in bone formation/resorption.

Question 9: Outline the mechanisms by which PTH exerts its effects on osteoclast bone resorption.

Question 10: Explain the metabolic significance of plasma alkaline phosphatase and osteocalcin levels.

Question 11: Outline the second messenger pathways that are believed to be involved in mediating the effects of PTH.

Question 12: Explain the source and physiological significance of the PTH-related protein (PTHrP).

Question 13: Describe the causes, symptoms and treatment of (a) hyperparathyroidism, (b) hypoparathyroidism. What are Chvostek's and Trousseau's signs?

Question 14: State the location of the parafollicular C cells, name their principal hormone secretion and give its effect on the plasma Ca^{2+} level.

Question 15: Describe the mechanisms regulating calcitonin release.

Question 16: Describe the main actions of calcitonin on (a) bone, (b) kidney; contrast the physiological significance of calcitonin, compared with PTH or vitamin D in regulating blood calcium levels?

Question 17: Outline the therapeutic uses of calcitonin in the treatment of Paget's disease and severe hypercalcaemia.

Question 18: Explain (giving named examples) the use of bisphosphonates in the treatment of (a) Paget's disease, (b) postmenopausal osteoporosis, (c) tumour-induced hypercalcaemia of malignancy.

Question 19: State the two natural forms of vitamin D and give its main effects on the plasma Ca^{2+} level.

Question 20: Give the main dietary sources of vitamin D.

Question 21: Outline the synthesis of vitamin D_3 in the skin and its conversion in the liver and kidney to active calcitriol.

Question 22: Describe the main actions of calcitriol on the gastrointestinal tract, bone and kidney.

Question 23: Outline how calcitriol exerts its effects via genomic and non-genomic receptor mechanisms.

Question 24: Describe the causes, symptoms (in children and adults) and treatment of vitamin D deficiency.

Question 25: List some commonly used vitamin D supplement preparations.

Question 26: Explain why patients taking high doses of vitamin D preparations require regular monitoring of plasma Ca^{2+}.

Question 27: Describe the causes, symptoms and treatment of vitamin D excess (hypervitaminosis D).

Question 28:   Outline the role of vitamin D in keratinocyte differentiation; what is the therapeutic significance of this effect?
Question 29:   Explain how other hormones can affect calcium homeostasis.
Question 30:   Describe the main types of primary osteoporosis; list the causes, symptoms and risk factors associated with this disorder and outline the therapeutic options available for treatment.

Clinical Case Studies

Patient 1

A 71 year old male was admitted to the emergency room in a confused, semi-comatose state, with dehydration, fatigue and abdominal pain; no other obvious abnormalities were evident. His blood pressure was 144/68 mmHg and heart rate 68 beats/min. The patient had lost 20 lb (9 kg) in the last four months, and was losing appetite. A neoplastic process was suspected and work up begun. On initial screening, he was found to have a high serum calcium level. A tentative diagnosis of *humoral hypercalcaemia of malignancy (HHM)* was made, an endocrinology consultation was sought and further studies undertaken.

On laboratory investigation, his full blood count (FBC) and urinalysis were normal; however, total serum calcium was 17.8 mg/dl (normal 8.4–10.7 mg/dl: 2.2–2.67 mmol/l), phosphate was 2.1 mg/dl (normal 2.5–4.8 mg/dl: 0.8–1.5 mmol/l), and alkaline phosphatase was elevated to 180 U/ml (normal 25–115 U/ml). The serum level of immunoreactive parathyroid hormone (iPTH) was 348 pg/ml (normal <65 pg/ml), while the level of parathyroid hormone-related protein (PTHrP) was normal. A 24 hour urinary calcium (total) measurement gave 420 mg/24 hours (normal 100–300 mg/24 hours).

An ultrasound of the neck revealed a left inferior parathyroid adenoma.

Question 1:   What is the most probable diagnosis in this case?
Question 2:   What are the usual causes and symptoms of hypercalcaemia?
Question 3:   How would this patient be managed?

Answer   1:   This patient has *hyperparathyroidism* arising from a *primary parathyroid adenoma*. The resultant high blood levels of PTH are associated with *hypercalcaemia*, a low serum phosphate (*hypophosphataemia*) and an excessive urinary excretion of calcium (*hypercalciuria*) and phosphate (*phosphaturia*); elevated serum levels of alkaline phosphatase are also present, reflecting an increase in bone osteoclast activity. A normal level of PTHrP (secreted by lung or breast carcinomas) supports the diagnosis of primary hyperparathyroidism, rather than humoral hypercalcaemia of malignancy (HHM). The plasma concentration of calcium normally regulates PTH release by a negative feedback mechanism exerted directly at the level of the parathyroid glands. In patients with parathyroid adenomas, the normal feedback mechanism is absent, and an increased secretion of PTH is maintained despite an elevated blood calcium level.

Answer   2:   *Primary hyperparathyroidism* is the most common cause of hypercalcaemia, and subtotal parathyroidectomy is the preferred treatment. Other causes of hypercalcaemia include: drugs (thiazide diuretics, chronic lithium treatment), vitamin D intoxication, malignancy, granulomatous diseases (sarcoidosis, berylliosis [systemic poisoning following inhalation of Be-Cu alloy], tuberculosis), immobilization (in Paget's disease) or in hyperthyroidism, acromegaly or acute adrenal failure (hypoadrenalism).

The usual signs and symptoms of hypercalcaemia include: tiredness, lethargy, depression, insomnia, headaches, general muscle weakness, anorexia, nausea/vomiting, dehydration (due to excessive urine loss), increased gastric acid/pepsin secretion, renal or uretic colic due to calculi, hypertension, and ECG changes (shortened QT interval)/cardiac arrhythmias.

Answer   3:   Following diagnosis, the patient was provided with intravenous hydration therapy with normal saline (over 10 days), in conjunction with an intravenous bisphosphonate (*disodium pamidronate*) to reduce his serum calcium level; [more acute cases of hypercalcaemia might require the use of a loop diuretic (*frusemide*) to promote a more rapid renal calcium excretion]. Once hydration was achieved, the patient underwent surgery, where an adenoma weighing 1.7 g was removed from the left parathyroid gland. The patient remained eucalcaemic after surgery and was discharged home.

Patient 2

A 32 year old female underwent sub-total thyroidectomy for treatment of Graves' disease. On the second hospital day the patient was complaining of a tingling sensation in her fingertips, tingling and numbness around the mouth and lips, and cramps in her legs and hands. Laboratory studies had previously been unremarkable for any calcium deficiency. On examination, the patient was alert and oriented; her heart rate was 112 beats/min, and blood pressure (BP) 146/96 mmHg. During BP recording, the patients hand went into a spasm (*Trousseau's sign*). Her deep tendon reflexes were brisk. The remainder of the examination was unremarkable. Clinical examination was consistent with *hypocalcaemia* and blood samples were drawn for immediate calcium measurement.

Laboratory data indicated a serum calcium level of 6.5 mg/dl (normal 8.4–10.7 mg/dl), ionized calcium 2.3 mg/dl (normal 3.6–4.1 mg/dl), phosphate 4.9 mg/dl (normal 2.5–4.8 mg/dl), and alkaline phosphatase 68 U/ml (normal 25–115 U/ml). Other laboratory data were normal.

Question   1:   *What is the likely cause of the patients hypocalcaemia? What major symptoms would you associate with the condition?*
Question   2:   *How would this patient be managed?*

Answer   1:   *Hypocalcaemia* in adults is usually an acquired phenomenon. It may be secondary to absence of parathyroid hormone (PTH) secretion, or a functional resistance to PTH (as seen in magnesium deficiency-*hypomagnesaemia*). It may also arise from nutritional deficiency of vitamin D (or inadequate exposure to UV light), chronic malabsorption, chronic renal disease, infiltration of the parathyroids by tumours or in *haemochromatosis* [an inherited condition characterized by excess iron deposition in the liver and endocrine glands). In this patient, the most plausible diagnosis would be *surgical hypoparathyroidism* arising from an inadvertent removal of parathyroid tissue, leading to mild hypocalcaemia and hyperphosphataemia (due to increased renal phosphate absorption) with a normal alkaline phosphatase; a low or undetectable serum iPTH level would also be expected [a similar condition can arise following radioactive iodine treatment for Graves' disease].

The major symptoms of hypocalcaemia include: tingling and numbness of the fingers, muscle cramps/spasm of the extremities, laryngeal stridor (harsh inspiratory sound, caused by laryngeal spasm) and in severe cases, tetany or general convulsions. Positive Trousseau's sign (wrist spasm induced by sphygmomanometer cuff inflation) and Chvostek's sign (twitching of facial muscles on tapping facial nerve) may be present; ECG changes (prolonged QT interval) and cardiac failure may also occur. In chronic cases, there is loss of body hair, drying of the skin and possible development of cataracts.

Answer 2: On confirming the hypocalcaemia, the patient was treated with an intravenous infusion of *10% calcium gluconate* over 48 hours to normalize the serum calcium level, at which point she was stable enough to be placed on oral calcium and vitamin D supplements for long-term maintenance. Regular serum and 24 hour urinary calcium measurements were made over the next two months to check for supplement overdosage, with possible development of *hyper*calcaemia.

UK/USA Drugs — Trade names		
	UK	**USA**
Bisphosphonates		
Disodium etidronate	Didronel	Didronel
Disodium pamidronate	Aredia	Aredia
Sodium clodronate	Loron; Bonefos	
Sodium alendronate	Fosamax	Fosamax
Vitamin D analogues		
Alfacalcidiol	One-Alpha; Alfa D	
Calcitriol	Calcijex Rocaltrol	Calcijex Rocaltrol
Dihydrotachysterol	AT 10	DHT
Tacalcitol	Curatoderm ointment	
Calcipotriol (Calcipotriene)	Dovonex cream	Dovonex ointment
Calcitonin		
Calcitonin (porcine)	Calcitare	
Salcatonin (synthetic salmon calcitonin)	Miacalcic Calsynar	Miacalcin Calcimar
Loop diuretic		
Frusemide (furosemide)	Lasix	Lasix

References

Books

- **Arnaud CD.** (1994). The calciotropic hormones & metabolic bone disease. In *Basic & Clinical Endocrinology*, edited by FS Greenspan, JD Baxter, 4th ed. Appleton & Lange, Connecticut, pp. 227–306
- **Aurbach GD, Marx SJ, Spiegel AM.** (1992). Parathyroid hormone, calcitonin and the calciferols. In *Williams Textbook of Endocrinology*, edited by JD Wilson, DW Foster, 8th ed. WB Saunders Company, USA, pp. 1397–1476
- **Bikle DD.** (1989). Agents that affect bone mineral homeostasis. In *Basic and Clinical Pharmacology*, edited by BG Katzung. Appleton & Lange, Connecticut, pp. 531–544
- **Breslau NA.** (1988). Calcium homeostasis. In *Textbook of Endocrine Physiology*, edited by JE Griffin, SR Ojeda. Oxford University Press, New York, pp. 273–301
- **Chandrasoma P, Taylor CR.** (1991). The parathyroid glands. In *Concise Pathology*, 1st ed. Prentice-Hall, USA, pp. 856–863
- **Dollery C.** (1991). *Therapeutic Drugs*, Vol. 1, Churchill Livingstone, Chapters on Calcifediol, Calciferol, Calcitonin and Calcitriol, pp. C8–C28
- **Ganong WF.** (1995). Hormonal control of calcium metabolism & the physiology of bone. In *Review of Medical Physiology*, 17th ed. Appleton & Lange, Connecticut, pp. 352–364
- **Genuth SM.** (1993). Endocrine regulation of calcium and phosphate metabolism. In *Physiology*, edited by RM Berne, MN Levy, 3rd ed. Mosby-Year Book Inc, USA, pp. 876–896
- **Goodman HM.** (1988). Hormonal regulation of calcium homeostasis. In *Basic Medical Endocrinology*. Raven Press, New York, pp. 175–202
- **Hedge GA, Colby HD, Goodman RL.** (1987). Control of calcium and phosphate metabolism. In *Clinical Endocrine Physiology*. WB Saunders Co, Philadelphia, Chapter 16, pp. 355–376
- **Holick MF, Krane SM, Potts Jr JT.** (1987). Disorders of bone and mineral metabolism. In *Harrison's principles of internal medicine*, edited by E Braunwald, KJ Isselbacher *et al.*, 11th ed. McGraw-Hill, Inc, USA, Chapters 335–336, pp. 1857–1889
- **Junqueira LC, Carneiro J & Long, J.A.** (1986). Adrenals & other endocrine glands. In *Basic Histology*, 5th ed. Lange Medical Publications, Connecticut, pp. 446–467
- **Kumar PJ, Clark ML.** (1990). Skeletal endocrinology. In *Clinical Medicine*, 2nd ed. Bailliere Tindall, pp. 820–827
- **Marcus R.** (1996). Agents affecting calcification and bone turnover. In *Goodman & Gilman's The Pharmacological Basis of Therapeutics*, edited by JG Hardman, LE Limbird, A Goodman Gilman *et al.*, 9th ed., McGraw-Hill, USA, pp. 1519–1546
- **Marshall WJ.** (1988). Calcium, phosphate, magnesium and bone. In *Illustrated Textbook of Clinical Chemistry*. Gower Medical Publishing, pp. 189–206
- **Rang HP, Dale MM.** (1991). The endocrine system. Parathyroid hormone, vitamin D and bone mineral homeostasis. In *Pharmacology*, 2nd ed. Churchill Livingstone, pp. 522–531
- **Rodan GA, Rodan SB.** (1995). The cells of bone. In *Osteoporosis: Etiology, Diagnosis and Management*, edited by BL Riggs, LJ Melton III, 2nd ed. Lippincot-Raven Publishers, Philadelphia, pp. 1–39
- **Shoback D, Draper MW.** (1992). Calcium & bone metabolism. In *Handbook of Clinical Endocrinology*, edited by PA Fitzgerald, 2nd ed. Prentice-Hall, USA, pp. 288–351
- **Thomas JA, Keenan EJ.** (1986). Parathyroid hormone and calcitonin. In *Principles of Endocrine Pharmacology*. Plenum Medical Book Company, New York, pp. 93–109

Journal Articles

- **Adachi JD.** (1997). Corticosteroid-induced osteoporosis. *Am J Med Sci*, 313, 41–49
- **Alper J.** (1994). Boning up: newly isolated proteins heal bad breaks. *Science*, 263, 324–325
- **Adler RA, Rosen CJ.** (1994). Glucocorticoids and osteoporosis. *Endocrinol Metab Clin North Am*, 23, 641–654
- **Bikle DD, Pillai S.** (1993). Vitamin D, calcium, and epidermal differentiation. *Endocrine Rev*, 14, 3–19
- **Bouillon R, Okamura WH, Norman AW.** (1995). Structure-function relationships in the vitamin D endocrine system. *Endocrine Rev*, 16, 200–256
- **Brown EM, Gamba G** *et al.* (1993). Cloning and characterization of an extracellular Ca^{2+}-sensing receptor from bovine parathyroid. *Nature*, 366, 575–580
- **Compston JE.** (1992). HRT and osteoporosis. *Br Med Bull*, 48, 309–344
- **Compston JE, Cooper C, Kanis JA.** (1995). Bone densitometry in clinical practice. *Br Med J*, 310, 1507–1511
- **Davies G.** (1994). Keep osteoporosis at bay. *Hospital Pharmacy Practice*, (Feb. 1994), 70–71
- **Dempster DW, Lindsay R.** (1993). Pathogenesis of osteoporosis. *Lancet*, 341, 797–801
- **Eriksen EF, Colvard DS** *et al.* (1988). Evidence of estrogen receptors in normal human osteoblast-like cells. *Science*, 241, 84–86
- **Fleisch H.** (1991). Bisphosphonates. Pharmacology and use in the treatment of tumour-induced hypercalcaemic and metastatic bone disease. *Drugs*, 42, 919–944
- **Fordham J.** (1997). Paget's disease: diagnosis and successful treatment. *Prescriber*, 8(11), 27–31
- **Francis RM.** (1995). Oral bisphosphonates in the treatment of osteoporosis: a review. *Current Therap Res*, 56, 831–851
- **Fraser DR.** (1995). Vitamin D. *Lancet*, 345, 104–107
- **Horowitz MC.** (1993). Cytokines and estrogen in bone: anti-osteoporotic effects. *Science*, 260, 626–627
- **Hurwitz S.** (1996) Homeostatic control of plasma calcium concentration. *Crit Rev Biochem Molec Biol*, 31, 41–100

- **Isaia G, Mussetta M** *et al.* (1994). Metabolic markers for the early diagnosis of postmenopausal osteoporosis. *J Endocrinol Invest*, 17, 771–774
- **Jones G, Calverley MJ.** (1993). A dialogue on analogues. Newer vitamin-D drugs for use in bone disease, psoriasis, and cancer. *Trends Endocrinol Metab*, 4, 297–303
- **Komm BS, Terpening CM** *et al.* (1988). Estrogen binding, receptor mRNA, and biologic response in osteoblast-like osteosarcoma cells. *Science*, 241, 81–83
- **Lindsay R.** (1993). Prevention and treatment of osteoporosis. *Lancet*, 341, 801–805
- **Mundy G.** (1995). No bones about fluoride. *Nature Medicine*, 1, 1130–1131
- **Muff R, Fischer JA, Biber J, Murer H.** (1992). Parathyroid hormone receptors in control of proximal tubule function. *Annu Rev Physiol*, 54, 67–79
- **Nissenson RA, Huang Z, Blind E, Shoback D.** (1993). Structure and function of the receptor for parathyroid hormone and parathyroid hormone-related protein. *Receptor*, 3, 193–202
- **Orwoll ES, Klein RF.** (1995). Osteoporosis in men. *Endocrine Rev*, 16, 87–116
- **Philbrick WM, Wysolmerski JJ. Galbraith S** *et al.* (1996). Defining the roles of parathyroid hormone-related protein in normal physiology. *Physiol Rev*, 76, 127–173
- **Prince RL.** (1996). Practice guidelines for the treatment of osteoporosis. *Calcif Tissue Int*, 59 (Suppl 1), S20–S23
- **Ratcliffe WA.** (1992). Role of parathyroid hormone-related protein in lactation. *Clin Endocrinol*, 37, 402–404
- **Rizzoli R, Ammann P.** (1993). Non-surgical treatment of primary hyperparathyroidism. *Acta Endocrinol*, 129, 375–376
- **Slosman DO, Rizzoli R, Bonjour J-Ph.** (1995). Bone absortiometry: a critical appraisal of various methods. *Acta Paediatr Suppl*, 411, 9–11
- **Vanderschueren D, Bouillon R.** (1995). Androgens and bone. *Calcif Tissue Int*, 56, 341–346
- **Walters MR.** (1992). Newly identified actions of the vitamin D endocrine system. *Endocrine Rev*, 13, 719–764
- **Werhya G, Leclère J.** (1995). Paracrine regulation of bone remodeling. *Horm Res*, 43, 69–75
- **Whitfield JF, Morley P.** (1995). Small bone-building fragments of parathyroid hormone: new therapeutic agents for osteoporosis. *Trends in Pharmacol Sci*, 16, 382–386

Abbreviations

ABP	androgen binding protein		HHM	humoral hypercalcaemia of malignancy
ACE	angiotensin-converting enzyme		HLA	human leucocyte antigen
ACTH	adrenocorticotrophic hormone (corticotrophin)		hPL	human placental lactogen
ADH	antidiuretic hormone		HRT	hormone replacement therapy
AIDS	acquired immune deficiency syndrome		11-HSD	11-β-hydroxysteroid dehydrogenase
ANP	atrial natriuretic peptide		Hsp	heat shock protein
AP-1	activator protein-1		5-HT	5-hydroxytryptamine
AR	androgen receptor protein		ICAs	islet cell antibodies
AREs	androgen-responsive elements		IDDM	insulin-dependent diabetes mellitus
ATP	adenosine triphosphate		IGF	insulin-like growth factor
AVP	arginine vasopressin		IGF-1	insulin-like growth factor-1
BMPs	bone morphogenic proteins		IGFs	insulin-like growth factors
BMR	basal metabolic rate		IL	interleukin
BPH	benign prostatic hyperplasia		IP$_3$	inositol-1,4,5-trisphosphate
CaBP	calcium binding protein		IRMA	immunoradiometric assay
cAMP	cyclic 3′,5′-adenosine monophosphate		IRS-1	insulin receptor substrate-1
CgA	chromogranin A		IUD	intrauterine device
cGMP	cyclic 3′,5′-guanosine monophosphate		IVF	*in vitro* fertilization
CNS	central nervous system		LDL	low density lipoprotein
COC	combined oral contraceptive		LH	luteinizing hormone
CRH	corticotrophin releasing hormone		LHRH	luteinizing hormone releasing hormone
CSII	continuous subcutaneous insulin infusion		βLPH	β-lipotrophin
CT	calcitonin		LTFs	ligand-activated transcription factors
CTBP	cytosolic thyroid hormone binding protein		MHC	major histocompatability complex
DAG	diacylglycerol		MIS	müllerian inhibiting substance
DHEAS	dehydroepiandrosterone sulphate		MIT	monoiodotyrosine
DHT	5α-dihydrotestosterone		MR	mineralocorticoid receptor protein
DIT	diiodotyrosine		MSH	melanocyte stimulating hormone
EPO	erythropoietin		NIDDM	non-insulin-dependent diabetes mellitus
FSH	follicle stimulating hormone		OGTT	oral glucose tolerance test
GABA	γ-aminobutyric acid		1,25-(OH)$_2$D$_2$)	1α,25-dihydroxycalciferol
GH	growth hormone		1,25-(OH)$_2$D$_3$	1α,25-dihydroxycholecalciferol
GH	growth hormone (somatotrophin)		25-(OH)D$_3$	25-hydroxycholecalciferol
GHRH	growth hormone releasing hormone		OP-1	osteogenic protein-1
GIP	gastric inhibitory peptide		PAPP-A	pregnancy-associated plasma protein-A
GLUT4	glucose transporter protein-4		PID	pelvic inflammatory disease
GM-CSF	granulocyte macrophage-colony stimulating factor		PLA$_2$	phospholipase A$_2$
GnRH	gonadotrophin-releasing hormone		POC	progestogen-only contraceptive
GR	glucocorticoid receptor protein		POMC	preproopiomelanocortin
HbA$_{1C}$	glycosylated haemoglobin fraction		PRL	prolactin
hCG	human chorionic gonadotrophin		PST	pancreastatin
hCS	human chorionic somatomammotrophin		PTH	parathyroid hormone
HDL	high density lipoprotein		PTHrP	parathyroid hormone-related protein
hGH	human growth hormone		PVN	paraventricular nucleus

rhRlx	recombinant human relaxin	**tGLP-1**	truncated glucagon-like peptide-1
rHuEPO	recombinant human erythropoietin	**TNF**	tumour necrosis factor
RIA	radioimmunoassay	**TNF-α**	tumour necrosis factor-α
rT$_3$	reverse T$_3$	**TR**	thyroid hormone receptor protein
SHBG	sex hormone binding globulin	**TRAP**	thyroid hormone auxiliary protein
SON	supraoptic nucleus	**TREs**	thyroid hormone response elements
SP-1	pregnancy-specific beta 1-glycoprotein	**TRH**	thyrotrophin releasing hormone
SRIH	somatotrophin release inhibiting hormone	**TSH**	thyroid stimulating hormone (thyrotrophin)
SS	somatostatin	**TSI**	thyroid-stimulating immunoglobulin
T$_3$	triiodothyronine	**VDDR**	vitamin D-dependent rickets
T$_4$	thyroxine	**VDR**	vitamin D receptor protein
TBG	thyroxine binding globulin	**VIP**	vasoactive intestinal polypeptide
TGF-β	transforming growth factor-β		

UK/US Spelling

UK	USA
Amenorrhoea	Amenorrhea
Analogue	Analog
Chiropodist	Podiatrist
Diarrhoea	Diarrhea
Foetus, Foetal	Fetus, Fetal
Galactorrhoea	Galactorrhea
Goitre	Goiter
Haemoglobin	Hemoglobin
Haemorrhage	Hemorrhage
Hormone Replacement Therapy	Estrogen Replacement Therapy (ERT)
Hypo-(hyper-)cholesterolaemia	-cholesterolemia
Hypo-(hyper-)calcaemia	-calcemia
Hypo-(hyper-)phosphataemia	-phosphatemia
Hypo-(hyper-)glycaemia	-glycemia
Hyperlipidaemia	Hyperlipidemia
Myxoedema	Myxedema
Neurone(s)	Neuron(s)
Oedema	Edema
Oestradiol, Oestriol	Estradiol, Estriol
Oestrogen, Oestrone	Estrogen, Estrone
Proteinurea	Proteinuria
Stilboestrol	(Diethyl)stilbestrol
Sulphonylurea	Sulfonylurea
Tumour	Tumor

Index

ABP see Androgen binding protein
Acarbose, 75
ACE see Angiotensin-converting enzyme
Acetylcholine, in regulation of CRH release, 9
Acidosis, in diabetes, 67, 76, 78, 79, 81
Acne, androgens affecting development of, 87, 88, 89
Acromegaly, 10, 14, 15, 20
ACTH (Corticotrophin) *see* Adrenocorticotrophic hormone;
ACTH stimulation test (short), 32, 39
Activator protein-1 (AP-1), 30
Activin, 87
Addison's disease, 30, 39, 40
Adenohypophysis: *see also* Pituitary gland, 7
Adenomas,
    adrenal, 32, 36, 38, 41
    parathyroid, 114, 125
    pituitary, 12, 15, 19, 38, 66, 106
    thyroid, 52
Adenylate cyclase/cAMP system, 1, 4
ADH *see* Antidiuretic hormone; Vasopressin
Adipose tissue, insulin effects on, 60, 62
Adrenal androgens, 32, 33, 94
Adrenal cortex
    and angiotensin II, 34
    hormones secreted by, 25
    malfunctions of, 30–33, 36
Adrenal crisis, 32
Adrenal glands
    ACTH effects on, 26, 32
    androgen secretion by, 25
    carcinoma of, 32
    dexamethasone effect on, 33, 38
    foetal, 93, 94
    structure and function of, 25
Adrenal hyperplasia, congenital, 32
Adrenal medulla,
    hormones secreted by, 25
Adrenalectomy, effects of, 30
Adrenaline, 25, 29
    metabolites, 40
Adrenocortical hormones, 25
    anatomical considerations, 25
    biosynthesis of, 26
    actions, 26–30, 34
    anti-inflammatory activity, 28, 29
    deficiencies of, 30, 32, 36
    excess of, 32, 36

receptors, 30, 31, 34, 35
    structure of, 26, 27
    uses, 28, 29, 32
Adrenocortical hyperfunction, 32, 36, 38, 40
Adrenocortical insufficiency, 30, 32, 36, 39
Adrenocorticotrophic hormone (ACTH);
(Corticotrophin): 11, 26
    actions, 11, 26
    biosynthesis/release, 11–12
    glucocorticoid secretion affected by, 11, 26
    hypersecretion of, 12, 32
    insufficiency of, 12, 30
    stress affecting secretion of, 12, 30
β-Adrenoreceptor blockers,
    in hyperthyroidism, 51, 54
AIDS (acquired immune deficiency syndrome),
    and adrenal insufficiency, 30, 36
Albumin, glucocorticoid binding to, 26
Aldosterone, 33
    actions of, 34
    antagonists, 34, 36, 41
    control of release, 34
    hypersecretion, 36
    hyposecretion, 36, 39
    mechanism of action, 35
    secretion and angiotensin II, 34
Aldosteronism, 36
Aldosteronoma, 41
Alfacalcidiol, 120
Alkaline phosphatase, 113, 116, 118, 125, 126
Alpha (α) islet cells (glucagon-secreting), 59
Alpha (α)-MSH (melanocyte stimulating hormone), 7, 11, 12,
    32, 39
Amino acids
    and GH secretion, 15
    and glucagon secretion, 65
    and insulin secretion, 60
Amenorrhoea, 33, 37, 53 *see also* Menstruation
Aminoglutethimide, 33
    for cancer chemotherapy, 98
    for Cushing's disease, 33
Amiodarone,
    interference with thyroid function, 50, 52
Amylin (islet amyloid polypeptide; IAPP), 65
AMP, cyclic (cAMP), *see also* Adenylate cyclase/cAMP system,
    1, 4
Anabolic effects of androgens, 89

Anabolic steroids, 89, *see also* Androgens
Androgens (male sex hormones), 87–89
 actions, 87
 adrenal, 87, 93, 94
 biosynthesis and structure, 27, 85
 control of release, 86
 on breast cancer, 89
 preparations available, 88, 108
 receptors, 87, 88, 89
 side effects, 89
 uses, 89
Androgen-binding protein (ABP), 86
Androgen replacement therapy, 88–89, 106
 preparations for, 88
Androgen resistance, 88
Androstenedione, 32, 88
Angiotensin(s), 34–36, *see also* Renin-angiotensin system
Angiotensin receptors (AT_{I-IV}), 35
Angiotensin-converting enzyme (ACE), 34
ACE inhibitors, 35
Angiotensinogen, 34
ANP *see* Atrial natriuretic peptide
Anterior pituitary gland, 7
Anterior pituitary hormones, 7, 10–16
 hypothalamic control of, 8
Adenohypophyseal hormones, 7, 10–16
Anti-adrenal antibodies, 39
Anti-androgens, 89, 98, 108, *see also* Oestrogens
Antidiabetic drugs: *see* Oral hypoglycemic drugs
Antidiuretic hormone (ADH); arginine
 vasopressin; vasopressin, 16–17
  actions, 16
  and ACTH release, 16
  analogues, 17
  control of release, 16–17
  deficiency of, 17
  excess, 17, *see also* SIADH
  receptors, 16
  synthesis/transport of, 16
Anti-oestrogens, 98
 for breast cancer, 98
Anti-inflammatory action of glucocorticoids, *see* Adrenocortical
 hormones
Anti-progestogen, 101
Antithyroid drugs, 51, 56, *see also* Thioureas
AP-1 (activator protein-1), 30
Aqueous iodine solution, 51, *see also* Lugol's iodine
Arachidonic acid, 3, 29
Arginine vasopressin (AVP); vasopressin: *see* Antidiuretic
 hormone
Aromatase, in oestrogen synthesis, 27
Aromatase enzyme inhibitors, 33, 38, 98
 for breast/prostate cancer, 98
 for Cushing's disease, 33
ATP (adenosine triphosphate)
 potassium channels and, 60
Atrial natriuretic peptide (ANP), 17
Autocrine secretion, 66

Beclomethasone, 28
Benign prostatic hyperplasia (BPH), 89
Beta (β)-MSH (melanocyte stimulating hormone), 11, 12
Beta (β) islet cells (insulin-secreting), 59
Beta (β)-lipotrophin (β-LPH), 11
Betamethasone, 28
Basal metabolic rate (BMR) thyroid hormone effects on, 47
Beta (β)-endorphin, 11, 12
Biguanides, 75, *see also* Oral hypoglycemic drugs
Bisphosphonates, 128
 for Paget's disease of bone, 117
 for osteoporosis, 117, 123
Blastocyst, 90
'Block-and-replace' treatment for Graves' disease, 51
Blood-testis barrier, 86
Bone
 resorption of, 112, 113–116, 117–118, 121
 calcium and, 111, 112–118
 continual remodeling of, 113, 114
 fracture, in osteoporosis, 121, 122–123
 glucocorticoid effects on, 121, 122
 oestrogen effects on, 114, 121
Breast
 carcinoma of, 89, 95, 98, 100
  chemotherapy for, 89, 98
 oxytocin effects, 7, 17
 prolactin effects, 13
Breast milk,
 and prolactin, 13
 and oxytocin, 17
Bromocriptine, 13, 14, 16, 19, 21
 uses in the treatment of,
  acromegaly, 16
  hyperprolactinaemia, 14
"Buffalo hump", in Cushing's syndrome, 33
Buserelin, 8, 95, 98

C-peptide (connection peptide),
 in insulin structure, 59–60, 73
C_{18-21} steroids, 26
Cabergoline, 14
Calcitonin, 111, 115, 116–117
 actions, 116
 uses in the treatment of,
  hypercalcaemia, 115
  osteoporosis, 123
  Paget's disease, 117
 control of release, 116
Calcitonin gene-related peptides (CGRP), 65
Calciferol, 117, 118, 119, 120
Calcitriol, 120
Calcium (ions), 111
 abnormal levels of,
  in hypercalcaemia, 114, 115, 116, 117, 120, 125–126
  in hypocalcaemia, 115, 116, 126–127
 calcitonin and, 116
 hormonal control of, 111
 parathyroid hormone secretion and, 112

Calcium-binding proteins,   118
Calcium supplements
    therapeutic uses,   117, 118, 120, 122–123
cAMP,   1, 4
Canrenoate (potassium),   34
Captopril,   35
Carbimazole,   51
Chief cells in parathyroid gland,
    secretions of,   111, 112
Chlorpropamide,   75, 82
Cholecystokinin,   65, 66
Cholesterol, and synthesis of steroids,   26
Chorionic gonadotrophin, *see*
    Human chorionic gonadotrophin (hCG)
Chromaffin cells,   25
Chvostek's sign, in tetany,   115
Circadian rhythm,
    ACTH/glucocorticoid secretion affected by,   12, 26
CLIP (corticotrophin-like intermediate lobe peptide),   12
Colles' fracture, in osteoporosis,   122
Colloid, thyroglobulin and,   45, 46
Congenital adrenal hyperplasia,   32
Conn's syndrome,   36
Contraception,
    hormonal,   98, 99–100
    intrauterine,   101–103
    'morning after',   98
Contraceptive pills oral,   101
    combined (COC's),   99
    progestogen-only (POC),   99
Corpus luteum,
    in menstrual cycle,   90–93
    in pregnancy,   92–93
    and relaxin secretion,   93
Corticosteroids,   25, 28, 30, 33, *see also* Adrenocortical
    hormones; Glucocorticoids; Mineralocorticoids; Steroids:
        blood glucose, effects on,   26, 28, 30, 33, 38
        deficiency, effects of,   32, 36
        excess, effects of,   32–33, 36
        synthesis/release,   26, 34–36
Corticotrophin (ACTH): *see* Adrenocorticotrophic hormone
Corticotrophin-like intermediate lobe peptide (CLIP),   12
Corticotrophs,   8, 9
Corticotrophin releasing hormone (CRH); corticoliberin;
    corticotrophin releasing factor (CRF),   9, 13
Cortisol (hydrocortisone),   11–13, 26–33
    actions,   26, 28–30
    intracellular mechanism,   30, 31
Cortisone,   32, 34
Cretinism,   48, 50
Creutzfeldt-Jakob disease,   15
CRH (corticotrophin releasing hormone),   9, 13
    -stimulation test,   33
Cryptorchidism,   88
Cushing's disease,   32, 38
Cushing's syndrome,   32–33, 38
    pituitary gland tumours causing,   32
Cyclic 3',5'-adenosine monophosphate, (cyclic AMP; cAMP),
    1, 4

Cyclic 3',5'-guanosine monophosphate (cyclic GMP; cGMP),   3
Cyclo-oxygenase (COX),   29
Cyclopentanoperhydrophenanthrene nucleus of steroid
    hormones,   26
Cyproterone, anti-androgenic activity,   89
Cytokines,   29, 30

Dehydroepiandrosterone (DHEAS),   25, 33
Delta (δ) islet cells (somatostatin-secreting),   59
Demeclocycline,   17
Deoxycorticosterone,   33
Desmopressin,   17
Dexamethasone,   28, 33
Dexamethasone suppression test, for
    Cushing's syndrome,   33, 38
Diabetes insipidus,   17
Diabetes mellitus,   68–76
    acidosis in,   67, 73, 76, 78–79
    coma in,   67, 76
    glucose tolerance test in,   72
    ketosis in,   67, 76
    symptoms of,   67
    types of,   68–69
    treatment,   72–75
    long-term complications of,   69–70
Diacylglycerol (DAG), and hormone effects,   3
Diazoxide,   70
Diethylstilbestrol (DES),   98
Diet-induced thyroid disease (from ingestion goitrogens),   49
Dihydrotestosterone (DHT),   87–88
1,25-Dihydroxycholecalciferol (1,25-Dihydroxyvitamin D$_3$),   112,
    113, 114, 117–118, 119, 120–122
Direct negative feedback,   3
DIT (diiodotyrosine),
    in thyroid hormone synthesis,   46
Dopamine, prolactin secretion and,   13
    TSH secretion and,   11
Dopamine receptor agonists, (*bromocriptine, cabergoline,
    quinagolide*),
    for acromegaly,   16
    for hyperprolactinaemia,   14
Drugs, effects on
    adrenal steroidogenesis,   33
    oestrogen synthesis,   98
Drugs,
    effects on thyroid function,   51
    male sexual function,   89
    pancreatic function,   70
    tranquillizers, effects on the endocrine system,   13
Drug-induced hypothyroidism,   51
Dwarfism,
    associated with cretinism,   50
pituitary,   15
    Laron-type,   15

Ectopic secretion of ACTH,   12, 32
Enalapril,   35

Endocrine glands, location and principal secretions of,   2, 3
Endocrine hypertension,   40
Endocrine pancreas, secretions of,   59
Endocrine system, introduction,   1
Endocrine target cells,
    hormones that act on,   2
Endometrial (uterine) cycle,   90–91, 92
Endometriosis,   95–96, 99
Endometrium, carcinoma of,   96, 98, 99, 100
Endorphin(s),   11; *see also:* Beta-endorphin(s)
Epiphyses (bone),
    hormones affecting,   87, 94
Erythropoietin,   89
Estrogens, *see* Oestrogens
Ethinyloestradiol,   96, 98, 100, 101
Ethynodiol diaacetate,   98, 101
Etidronate,   117, 123
Exocrine glands, definition of,   1
Exophthalmos,   50

Familial glucocorticoid deficiency (FGD),   32
F islet cells, pancreatic,   59
Facial changes,
    and growth hormone excess,   15
    and thyroid hormones,   49, 50
Feedback control
    of hormone secretion,   3–5
Female hypogonadism,   95, 96, 106
Female reproductive system,   90–95
    hormonal control of uterine cycle,   90–92
    ovarian cycle and hormone release,   90
    structure,   90, 91
Female sex steroids: *see* Oestrogens
Finasteride,   89
Fludrocortisone,   32, 40
Fluocinolone,   28
Flutamide,   89
Fluoride, and osteoporosis,   123
Follicle,
    Graafian,   90, 91
    thyroid,   45
Follicle stimulating hormone (FSH),
    in females,   10, 90–92, 93–94, 95, 98, 99, 106
    in males,   10, 86–87
Follicular cells (in thyroid),   45–47, 105
Follicular development and regression,
    during menstrual cycle,   90–92
Follistatin,   87
Frusemide,   40–41, 115, 126

G-protein(s),
    hormone receptors coupled to,   4
GABA (γ-aminobutyric acid),   9, 13
Galactorrhoea,   13, 18
Gamma (γ)-lipotrophin,   11, 12
Gastric inhibitory peptide (GIP),   60, 66

Gastrin,   60, 66
Gastrin-releasing peptide (GRP),   66
Gastrinoma,   66
Gastrointestinal hormones,   66–67
    effects on glucagon secretion,   65
    effects on insulin secretion,   60
Gestational diabetes,   69
Gigantism, pituitary,   15
Glibenclamide (glyburide),   75, 82
Gliclazide,   75, 82
Glipizide,   75, 82
Gliquidone,   75
Glucagon,   59, 64–65, 66, 67
    actions,   69, 65
    synthesis/release,   64–65
    and insulin-glucagon molar ratio,   65
Glucocorticoids,   25–33, *see also* Adrenocortical hormones;
        Corticosteroids; Steroids:
    actions,   26–30
    anti-allergic effects,   29
    as anti-inflammatory agents,   28–29
    as antirheumatoid agents,   28
    as immunosuppressants,   29–30
    control of release,   26
    effects on blood glucose,   26, 28, 33, 38
    effects on bone calcium metabolism,   32–33, 121
    excess of,   32–33
    in Cushing's syndrome,   32–33, 37–38
    insufficiency of,   30, 32
    intracellular mechanism of action,   30–31
    preparations,   28, 42
    receptors,   30–31
    and resistance to "stress",   30
Glucocorticoid receptor protein (GR),   30–31
Glucocorticoid response elements (GREs),   30–31
Gluconeogenesis, hormones affecting,   62, 63, 65
Glycogenolysis, hormones affecting,   62, 63, 65
Glucose,
    blood level of,   67, 79
    glucagon secretion affected by,   65
    insulin secretion affected by,   60
    renal threshold for,   67
    -suppression test for acromegaly,   16
    tests for,   70, 71
    -tolerance test (oral), for diabetes,   72, 80–81
Glycolysis, insulin effects,   62
Glycosuria,   67
Glycosylated haemoglobin (HbA),   70, 78–79
Glyburide (Glibenclamide),   75, 82
GnRH-associated peptide (GAP),   9
Goitre,   49, 50, 52
    toxic multinodular,   52
Goitrogens,   49
Gonad(s), malfunctions of,   88, 95, 105–106
Gonadal hormones and reproduction,   85
Gonadorelin,   8–9
Gonadotrophin(s),   10, 86, 88, 90–92, 94, 105–106;
    see also Follicle-stimulating hormone;

Luteinizing hormone
Gonadotrophin releasing hormone (GnRH);
    Luteinizing hormone releasing hormone (LHRH)
        analogues of, 8–9, 95, 98
Gonadotrophin release inhibitors, 95
Gonadotrophs, 8–9
Goserelin, 95, 98
Graafian (ovarian) follicle, 90–91
Granulocyte macrophage colony stimulating factor (GM-CSF),
    29, 113, 114, 121
Granulosa cells,
    and oestrogen secretion, 90
    and inhibin production, 91
Graves' disease, 50, 53–54
Growth factors *see* Insulin-like growth factors
Growth hormone (GH), 14–16; *see also*
    Somatotrophin
        actions, 14
        clinical use, 15
        control of release, 14–15
        deficiency of, 15
        diabetogenic effect of, 14
        excess, 15–16
        human (somatropin), 15
Growth hormone releasing hormone (GHRH);
    somatocrinin, 9–10, 14–15
Growth hormone release-inhibiting hormone, *see*
    Somatostatin
Guar Gum, 75
Guanine nucleotide regulatory protein(s), *see*
    G-protein(s)
Guanylate cyclase, 3
Guanosine diphosphate (GDP), 4
Guanoside triphosphate (GTP), 4
Gut glucagon, 64

Haloperidol, 13
Hashimoto's thyroiditis, 49
Heat shock protein(s) (Hsp), 30, 31
Hexarelin, 9
    HDLs (high-density lipoproteins), 96
Hirsutism, 3.3, 37–38
HLA system, and susceptibility to diabetes, 68–69, 78–79
Homeostasis, plasma calcium, 112, 113, 116–118, 121
Hormone(s); *see also specific types*:
    communication, 1, 3
    definition of, 1
    feedback mechanisms, 3–5
    mechanisms of action, 1, 3
    of endocrine system, 2
    of gastrointestinal tract (endocrine), 66–67
    response elements, 1, 3, 30–31, 48, 87
    steroid, 1, 26, 85, 87, 93, 94–95
    thyroid, 45–49
    types of, 1
Hormone receptors (types of), 1, 3, 4
Hormone replacement therapy (HRT), 96–97, 101, 102

Hormone-sensitive lipase, 62, 64, 65, 68
5-HT (serotonin),
    in regulation of CRH release, 9
Human chorionic gonadotropin (hCG), 92–93, 103, 106
Human insulin, 73, 74, 82
Human leucocyte antigens (HLA),
    and diabetes, 68–69, 78–79
Human menopausal gonadotropins (hMG), 94, 106; *see also*
    Menotrophin
Human placental lactogen (hPL), 93
Humoral hypercalcaemia of malignancy (HHM), 114, 117, 125
Humulin (human insulin), 73, 74, 82
Hydrocortisone, 29, 32, 40; *see also* Cortisol
25-hydroxycholecalciferol (25-Hydroxyvitamin D_3), 118, 119, 120
11β-Hydroxylase, in steroid synthesis, 33
21β-Hydroxylase, in steroid synthesis, 32
11β-hydroxysteroid dehydrogenase, 34
Hyperaldosteronism,
    primary (Conn's syndrome), 36, 40
    secondary, 36
Hypercalcaemia
    effects of, 115, 125–126
    in hyperparathyaroidism, 114–115, 125–126
    treatment, 115, 117, 125–126
Hypercortisolism, 32, 33; *see also* Cushing's Syndrome
Hyperglycaemia,
    effects of, in diabetes, 67
    in Cushing's syndrome, 33
    management of (diabetes), 72–75
Hyperinsulinism, 69, 70
Hyperparathyroidism, 114–115, 125–126
Hyperphosphataemia, 115, 126
Hyperpituitarism; *see individual pituitary hormones*
Hyperprolactinaemia, 13, 18–19
Hyperthyroidism (thyrotoxicosis), 50–52
    basal metabolic rate (BMR) and, 50
    causes of, 50, 52
    drugs used in treatment, 51, 56
    main symptoms of, 50, 52, 53–54
    secondary, 52
    TRH test for, 52
Hypervitaminosis D, 120
Hypoaldosteronism, 36
Hypoadrenalism, 30, 32, 39; *see also* Addison's disease
Hypocalcaemia,
    tetany from, 115
Hypoglycaemia, 75–76
    due to insulin excess, 70, 75
    symptoms of, 76
    treatment, 76
Hypoglycaemic drugs, oral, 74–75, 82
Hypogonadism, 88, 95
Hypokalaemia, 36, 40
Hypoparathyroidism, 115–116, 120, 126–127
Hypophosphataemia, 114, 125
Hypopituitarism, 15, 20
Hypothalamic-hypophyseal portal system, 8
Hypothalamohypophyseal tract, 16

Hypothalamus, 7
  hormones secreted by, 8–10
  feedback effects on, 3–5
Hypothyroidism, 49–50
  childhood (congenital), 50
  drug therapy, 49–50
  main symptoms of, 49–50
  tests for, 49–50

^{131}I (radioactive iodine), 51
Immunoglobulins, thyroid-stimulating, 50, 54
Immunosuppression,
  by corticosteroids, 29–30
Implants (subcutanaeous),
  of progestogens, 99
Indirect negative feedback, 4–5
Inflammatory response, inhibition
  by corticosteroids, 28–29
Inhibin, 10, 86–87, 91–92
Inositol (1,4,5)-trisphosphate (IP$_3$),
  and mediation of hormone effects, 34, 35
Insulin, 59–64
  actions, 60–62
  deficiency of, 67–69; see also Diabetes mellitus
  effects on glucose transporter proteins, 61–62
  enzymes affected by, 63, 64
  excess, 69, 70
  -glucagon molar ratio, 65
  human, 73, 74, 82
  injection pens, 72
  mechanism of action, 63–64
  metabolic effects of, 60–63
  mixtures of, 73–74, 82
  pumps, 72
  receptor, 63–64
  receptor substrate-1 (IRS-1), 64
  resistance, 69, 75
  preparations, 73–74, 82
  synthesis/secretion, 59–60, 61
  structure, 59
  and sulphonylureas,
    combined therapy with, 80
  -tolerance test, 15
  treatment with, 72–74
Insulin-dependent diabetes mellitus (IDDM; Type diabetes
  mellitus), 68
Insulin-like growth factors (IGFs; Somatomedins), 14–15,
  19–20, 64
  and GH release, 15
  receptors for, 64
Insulin lispro, 73–74
Insulinoma, 70
Intrauterine devices (IUDs), 101–103
  progestogen-impregnated, 102–103
Interferon-γ, 29
Interleukins (ILs), 13, 29, 113, 114, 121
Interstitial cells of Leydig, 10, 86–88

Iodination of thyroglobulin, 45–47
Iodine (iodide)
  and thyroid gland, 46–47
  use in hyperthyroidism, 51
  radioactive, uses, 51
Iodine deficiency goitre, 50
Islet amyloid polypeptide (IAPP), see Amylin
Islets (pancreatic) of Langerhans, 59
Islet cell,
  antibodies (ICAs), 68
  tumour of (insulinoma), 70
  transplants, 73
Islet cells (pancreatic), hormones secreted by, 59

Juxtaglomerular cells, renin secretion by, 34

Ketone bodies (in diabetes), tests for, 70, 78
Ketosis (ketoacidosis), diabetic, 67, 76, 78–79

Lactation,
  secretion and ejection of milk, 13, 17
Laron dwarfism, 15
LDL (low-density lipoprotein)-cholesterol, 48, 87, 96
Levonorgestrel, 98–102
Lente insulin, 74, 82
Leuprorelin, 8, 95, 98
Leydig, interstitial cells of, 10, 86–88
Liothyronine, (Levothyroxine sodium), 49, 56
Lipodystrophy, insulin-induced, 72
Lipolysis, hormones affecting, 28, 48, 62, 65, 68
Lithium carbonate,
  and thyroid hormone release, 49
Losartan, 36
Lugol's iodine solution, 51
Luteinizing hormone (LH), 10, 11, 18–20, 86, 90–95, 99,
  105–106
  preovulatory surge of, 90–92
Luteinizing hormone releasing hormone (LHRH),
  see Gonodotrophin releasing hormone
Lymphokines, 29
Lypressin, 17

Male hypogonadism, 88, 105–106
  treatment of, 88–89, 105–106
Male reproductive system, 85–89
  hormonal control of, 86–87
  endocrine function of, 85
Mammary gland, see Breast
Major histocompatability complex, 68
Median eminence, 8
Medroxyprogesterone, 96, 98–100, 102
Medullary carcinoma of thyroid,
  calcitonin excess in, 116
Melanocyte stimulating hormone(s) (MSH), 7, 11, 12, 32

Menopause, symptoms of, 93–94, 96
    hormone replacement therapy (HRT) and, 96–97, 100–101
  osteoporosis and, 93–94, 121–122
Menotrophin (human menopausal gonadotrophins; hMG),
    94, 106
Menstrual cycle
    hormonal control of, 91–92
Menstruation
    cessation of (amenorrhoea), 32, 33, 37–39, 53
Mesterolone, 89
Mestranol, 96, 100, 101
Metformin, 75, 82
Metyrapone, 33
Methimazole, 51
Methyltestosterone, 89, 108
Microadenoma, 32, 38
Mifepristone, 101
Milk, *see also* Breast milk,
    inappropriate production of (galactorrhoea), 13, 18–19
    let-down, 17
    oxytocin and, 17
    secretion and ejection of, 13, 17
Mineralocorticoids, 33–36; *see also*
    Corticosteroids; Steroids:
        actions, 34
        control of release, 34–36
        deficiency, effects of, 36
        excess, effects of, 36
        mechanism(s) of action, 34
        receptors, 34, 35
Mineralocorticoid receptor protein (MR), 34, 35
Mini-pumps for insulin delivery, 72–73
MIT (monoiodotyrosine), 46–47
"Moon face", in Cushing's syndrome, 33, 37–39
"Morning after" contraceptive pill, 98
α/β-MSH, *see* Melanocyte-stimulating homone
Müllerian inhibiting substance (MIS), 88
Multiple endocrine neoplasia (MEN-1 disease);
    (Multiple endocrine adenomatosis; MEA), 114–115
Myoepithelial cells, oxytocin effects on, 17
Myxoedema, and hypothyroidism, 49, 54–55

Nadolol, 51
Nafarelin, 8, 95
Nandrolone, 89
Natriuretic peptide, atrial, *see* Atrial natriuretic peptide (ANP)
Nelson's syndrome, 12
Negative feedback inhibition, 3–5
Neurogenic feedback (during suckling), 13–14, 17
Neurohypophysis: *see* Pituitary gland, 7, 16
Neurohypophyseal hormones (posterior
    pituitary hormones), 16–17
Neuropeptide Y (NPY), 66
Neurophysins, for oxytocin and vasopressin, 16
Neurotensin, 66
Non-insulin dependent diabetes mellitus (NIDDM; Type 2
    diabetes mellitus), 68–69

Noradrenaline, 25
Noradrenaline metabolites, 40
Norethisterone, 96, 98–102
Norgestrel, 98, 100, 102

Octreotide, 10, 16, 19–21
Oestradiol, 85–86, 92–94, 96, 97, 100, 102, 108
    binding to plasma proteins, 94
    structure of, 85
Oestradiol valerate, 96, 97, 102
Oestriol, 92, 94, 96, 97, 102
Oestrogens (female sex hormones); Estrogens:
    actions, 5, 94
    biosynthesis of by granulosa cells, 90
    and bone mineral homeostasis, 93–94, 96, 114, 121–123
    in HRT preparations, 96–97, 100–102
    natural, 96–97
    and progestogens, combinations of (for contraception),
        89, 101
    receptors, 95
    uses, 96–102
Oestrone, 92, 93–94, 96–97
Oral contraceptives, 98, 99–101; *see also* Oestrogens;
    Progestogens:
    mechanism of action, 98, 99
    preparations, 101
    side effects, 99, 100
Oral glucose tolerance test, 72, 80–81
Oral hypoglycaemic drugs, 74–75, 82
Osteoblasts, deposition of bone by, 113, 114, 116–118, 121, 123
Osteoclasts, bone calcium mobilization by, 113, 114, 116–118,
    121, 122
Osteocytes, formation of, 113
Osteomalacia, 118, 120
Osteopenia, 19, 121
Osteoporosis, 117, 118, 121–123
    bisphosphonates for, 123
    calcitonin for, 123
    glucocorticoid-induced, 121
    oestrogens for (HRT), 96–97, 102, 123
Ovarian cycle, and hormone release, 90–92
    follicular development during, 90, 91
    hormonal regulation of, 92
    luteal phase of, 90–92
Ovarian follicle, 90–93
Ovarian hormones, 90–93; *see also* Oestrogens; Progesterone
Ovary,
    tumours of, 95
    structure, 90–91
Ovulation, 90–92
    luteinizing hormone in, 90–92
    menstrual cycle and, 91
Ovulation-inducing agents, 92, 94, 98
Oxyphil cells, in parathyroid gland, 111
Oxytocin, 7, 9, 16, 17
    actions, 17
    clinical uses, 17

control of release,   17
in parturition,   17
in prolactin release,   13
synthesis/transport,   16

Paget's disease of bone,   116–117
Pancreas, endocrine secretions of,   59–67
Pancreastatin,   66
Pancreatic islets of Langerhans, hormones
    produced by,
        glucagon,   64–65
        insulin,   59–64
        miscellaneous,   65–67
Pancreatic polypeptide,   59, 66
Panhypopituitarism,   15
Paracrine (hormone) action,   1, 10, 59, 66, 86, 87, 114, 118, 121
Parafollicular cells, calcitonin secretion by,   45, 116
Parathyroid glands,
    structure of,   111
    inadvertent removal of,   52, 115, 126–127
Parathyroid hormone (PTH),   111–116
    actions of,   112–114
    control of release,   112
    cyclic AMP and,   113
    deficiency,   115–116, 126–127
    excess,   14–115, 125–126
Parathyroid hormone-related protein (PTHrP),   114
Parathyroidectomy, effects of,   115, 126–127
Paraventricular nucleus (oxytocin secretion by),   16, 17
Pars distalis,   7
Pars intermedia,   7, 11, 12
Pars nervosa,   7
Peptide YY (PYY),   66
Perchlorate,   46
Pertechnetate,   46
Phaeochromocytoma,   40
Phosphate,   111–116, 117–118, 125–127
    abnormal levels of,   114, 115
    in hypercalcaemia,   114, 125–126
Phosphatidylinositol metabolism
    and hormone action,   3, 16, 17, 113
Phosphodiesterase, cAMP hydrolysis by,   4
Phospholipase A_2 (PLA$_2$)
    glucocorticoid inhibition by,   29
Phospholipase C, activation by hormone action,   35
Phosphorylation
    of insulin receptor,   63–64
    of key enzymes (and insulin action),   64
Pituicytes,   16
Pigmentation (skin), agents affecting,   7, 11–12, 32
Pituitary gland,
    anterior (adenohypophysis),   7
    hyperfunction,   10–16
    insufficiency,   10–16
    microadenomas of,   12, 18–19, 32, 38
    posterior (neurohypophysis),   7, 16
    structure of,   7
Pituitary hormones,

    anterior,   10–16
    posterior,   16–17
Pituitary function tests,   8, 15–16
Pituitary gonadotrophins, *see* Gonadotrophins
Placenta, endocrine secretions of,   10, 92–94
Placental lactogen, *see* Human placental lactogen
Polydipsia,
    in Cushing's syndrome,   33
    in diabetes mellitus,   67
    in diabetes insipidus,   17
Polyuria,
    in Cushing's syndrome,   33
    in diabetes insipidus,   17
    in diabetes mellitus,   67
Positive feedback,   5, 91–92
    short-loop,   5, 14, 15
Postcoital contraception, "morning after pill",   98
Posterior pituitary gland,   7, 16
Posterior pituitary hormones,   16–17
    see also Neurohypophyseal hormones
Postmenopausal women, hormone replacement therapy (HRT)
    for,   96–97, 101, 102
Potassium (ions),
    and aldosterone secretion,   36
Potassium channels, ATP-sensitive,   60–61, 74
Potassium iodide tablets,   51
Precocious puberty,   10, 88
Prednisolone,   28
Pregnancy,
    -associated plasma protein-A (PAPP-A),   93
    foetal-placental unit and,   93, 94
    hormonal changes during,   92–93
    placental hormones,   92–94
    testing,   103
Pregnant mare urine (conjugated oestrogens from),   96, 97, 102
Preproglucagon,   60, 64
Preproinsulin,   59
Preproopiomelanocortin (POMC),   11–12
Primordial (ovarian) follicle,   90–91
Progesterone,   10, 85, 90–96, 100–101
    actions,   94–95
    in menstrual cycle,   90–92
    receptors,   95
    secretion,   90–92
Progestogens,   85, 94–96, 98–103, 108
    combined with oestrogens (for contraception),   99–101
    preparations,   96, 98–103, 108
    uses,   98–103
Proinsulin,   14, 59
Prolactin (PRL),   13–14
    actions,   13
    control of release (dopamine and),   13, 14
    drugs affecting secretion,   13, 14
    excess of,   13–14, 18–19
Prolactin releasing/inhibiting factors,   9–10, 14
Prolactinoma,   13
Proliferative phase of menstrual cycle,   90
Propranolol,   51
Propylthiouracil,   51

Prostaglandins, 3, 29
Prostaglandin synthesis (inhibition of), 29
Prostate, benign hyperplasia of (BPH), 89
Protein anabolic steroids (androgens), 87, 89
Protein kinase(s)
    and insulin action, 63–64
Protein kinase A, 4
Protein kinase C, 3
Protirelin (synthetic TRH), 9
Pseudohypoparathyroidism, 115
PTH,
    and vitamin D, interaction of, 112, 115, 119
Pumps, for insulin delivery, 72–73

Quinagolide, 14

Radioactive iodine (¹³¹I),
    and thyroid gland, 51, 52
Receptors (hormone), and signal transduction mechanisms,
    1, 2, 4
5-α-Reductase, 87
    deficiency, 88
    inhibitor, 89
Relaxin, 93
Releasing hormones (hypothalamic), 8–10
Renin,
    secretion, 34
    hypersecretion, 36
Renin-angiotensin (-aldosterone) system, 34
Reproductive organs, effects of sex steroids, 87, 94
Retinoic acid, 30
Reverse T₃ (rT₃), 46, 48, 50, 52
    structure of, 46
Rheumatoid arthritis, glucocorticoids in, 28
Rickets
    nutritional, 118, 120
    vitamin D-dependent (type 1), 118
    vitamin D-dependent (type 2), 120

Sodium (ions),
    retention, hormones causing, 34, 36, 40–41, 89, 99, 100
Salcatonin, 115, 117, 123
Saline diuresis, in hypercalcaemia, 115, 126
Sarcoidosis, 120, 125
Schwartz-Bartter Syndrome, 17; see also
    Syndrome of inappropriate ADH (SIADH)
Second messenger systems, 1
Secondary diabetes, 68
Secondary hypoadrenalism, 32
Secondary (ovarian) follicles, 90, 91
Secretin, 60, 66
Selective oestrogen receptor modulator (SERM), 123
Sermorelin, 9
Serotonin (5-hydroxytryptamine; 5-HT), 9, 13
Sertoli cells, 10, 86

Sex characteristics,
    oestrogens affecting (female), 94
    testosterone affecting (male), 87
Sex hormone-binding globulin (SHBG), 87, 94
Sex steroids, 25, 85
SH2 domain proteins, 64
Short-acting insulin, 74
'Short-loop' feedback, 5
'Sick euthyroid' syndrome, 52
Skin,
    and oral contraceptives, 100
    and thyroid hormones, 48–50, 54–55
Sodium
    and water, balance of, effects of mineralocorticoids, 34
Somatomedins, 14, 15; see also: Insulin-like
    growth factors (IGFs),
        and GH release, 15
Somatostatin (SS); Somatotrophin-release
    inhibiting hormone (SRIH), 10, 11, 15, 16, 19–21, 59, 60,
        65, 66
            actions, 10
            analogue, 10, 16, 21
            and GH release, 14–15
            clinical uses, 10, 16, 21
            and TSH secretion, 11
Somatotrophin (GH; growth hormone),
    actions, 14
    clinical use, 15
    control of release, 14–15
    deficiency of, 15
    diabetogenic effect of, 14
    excess, 15–16
    human (somatropin), 15
Somatotrophs, 8
Somatropin, 15
Sotalol, 51
Spermatogenesis, control of, 86
Spironolactone, 34, 36, 41
Src-homology 2 (SH2) protein domain, 64
Stanozolol, 89
Steroid(s)/steroid hormone(s), 1, 3, 26, 27, 30–31, 85–87,
        94–95, 117–119; see also
    Glucocorticoids; Mineralocorticoids; Vitamin D:
        adrenal, see Corticosteroids
        anabolic, 89
        anti-inflammatory action, 29
        receptors, 30–31, 34–35, 87–88, 95, 118
        synthesis inhibitor drugs, for cancer chemotherapy, 98
        -treatment cards, 30
Steroid-carrying plasma proteins, 26, 87, 94, 95, 118
Stilboestrol, 97–98
Stones, renal, and hyperparathyroidism, 115
Stress,
    and ACTH/cortisol secretion, 12, 13, 30
    and GH secretion, 14–16
    and prolactin secretion, 13–14
    glucocorticoids affecting resistance to, 30
Striae (abdominal), in Cushing's syndrome, 33
Sulphonylureas, 74–75, 82; see also Oral

hypoglycaemic drugs,
potassium channels and, 61, 74
Subcutaneous implants, *see* Implants
Supraoptic nucleus (ADH secretion by), 7, 16
Syndrome of inappropriate hypersecretion of ADH (SIADH), 17

T_3 (triiodothyronine), and T_4, (tetraiodothyronine; thyroxine),
10, 11, 45–52, 53–55
Tamoxifen,
for breast cancer, 98
TBG (thyroxine-binding globulin), 46, 52
Testes, 85–89
-blood barrier and, 86
endocrine function of, 87
hyperfunction, 88
hypofunction, 88, 105–106
structure, 85–86
undescended (cryptorchidism), 88, 92
Testosterone, 85–88; *see also* Androgens
actions, 87
baldness and, 87
clinical uses, 88–89
control of release, 10–11, 86–87
mechanism of action, 87–88
preparations, 88, 108
structure, 85
Tetany, in hypocalcaemia, 115, 126–127
Testosterone enanthate, 88
Testosterone proprionate, 88
Testosterone undecanoate, 88
Tetracosactrin, 11, 32, 39–40
Thiazolidinediones, 75
Thiocyanate, 46
Thiourea derivatives (thionamides), 51
Thyroglobulin, 10, 45–47
Thyroid gland, 45
and antithyroid drugs, 51, 56
and beta-blockers, 51
carcinoma of (follicular type), 52
dysfunction, 49–52
function, control of hormone release, 10–11, 47
medullary carcinoma of, 116
structure, 45
Thyroid function tests, 53–54
Thyroid hormone(s), *see* T_3/T_4
actions, 47–49
receptor mechanisms, 48–49
structure, 46
synthesis, 46–47
transport of, 46
control of release, 10–11, 47
Thyroid stimulating hormone (TSH;
thyrotrophin), 3–4, 10–11, 46–47, 49–50, 52, 53–55
Thyroid-stimulating immunoglobulins (TSIs), 50, 53–54
Thyroid storm, 52
Thyroidectomy, 51–52
Thyroiditis, subacute, 52
Thyroid-pituitary relationships, 11, 47

Thyrotoxic crisis, 51, 52
Thyrotoxicosis, *see also* Hyperthyroidism
effects of, 50
factitia, 52
treatment, 51
Thyrotrophin (TSH): *see* Thyroid stimulating hormone
Thyrotrophin releasing hormone (TRH), 9–11, 13, 14, 47, 52
Thyrotrophs, 8
Thyroxine (*L-thyroxine sodium*)
actions, *see* T_4
-binding globulin (TBG), 46, 52
-binding prealbumin, 46
biosynthesis/secretion, 45–47
control of release, 47
structure, 46
uses, 49–50
TNF-α: *see* Tumour necrosis factor-α
Tolazamide, 75, 82
Tolbutamide, 75–82
Toxic multinodular goitre, 52
Toxic nodule (solitary), 52
Transcalciferin, 118
Transcortin, 26
Transforming growth factor-β (TGF-β), 88, 121
TRH test, 52
Triamcinolone, 28
Trifluoperazine, 13
Tri-iodothyronine (*liothyronine*),
actions, *see* T_3
receptors for, 48–49
secretion, 47
structure, 46
3,3′,5′-Triiodothyronine (T_3), structure of, 46
3,5,3′-Triiodothyronine (rT_3), structure of, 46
Troglitazone, 75
Trophic hormone(s), 3–5, 7, 10–16
Trousseau's sign, in tetany, 115, 126–127
Truncated glucagon-like peptide (tGLP-1), 60
Tumour necrosis factor-α, 13, 29, 121
Turner's syndrome, 95
Type 1 diabetes mellitus: *see* Insulin-dependent diabetes mellitus (IDDM)
Type 2 diabetes mellitus: *see* Non-insulin dependent diabetes mellitus (NIDDM)
Tyrosine derivatives, iodination of, and thyroglobulin, 46, 47

Ultralente insulin, 82
Urine, glucose tests of, 70, 78
Uterus
and oral contraceptives, 99–100
endometrial cancer of, 98, 99, 100
oxytocin stimulation by, 17

Valsartan, 36
Vasoactive intestinal polypeptide (VIP), 66, 67
Vasopressin: *see* Antidiuretic hormone (ADH)
Verner-Morrison Syndrome, 67

Virilization,
    21β-hydroxylase enzyme deficiency and, 32
    in Cushing's syndrome, 33
5-α-reductase deficiency and, 88
Vitamin D, 111–114, 116, 117–121
    actions, 118, 120
    analogues, 120, 128
    and PTH, interaction of, 112, 113, 118, 119
    deficiency, 118, 120
    excess (hypervitaminosis D), 120
    malabsorption/deficiency and hypocalcaemia, 118, 126–127
    metabolism, 113, 117–119
    receptors(VDRs) for, 118
    structure, 119
Vitamin D-binding globulin (transcalciferin), 118
Vitamin D-dependent rickets (type 1), 118
Vitamin D-dependent rickets (type 2), 120
Vitamin D_2 (ergocalciferol), 117–120

Vitamin D_3 (cholecalciferol), 117–120
VMA (vanillylmandelic acid), 40

Water (fluid) excretion of, hormones affecting, **16–17, 33–36**
Weight gain, due to oral contraceptives, 99, 100
Withdrawal bleeding,
    in oral contraception, 99, 100
    in HRT, 100, 101

Zinc, insulin preparations containing, **73, 74**
Zollinger-Ellison syndrome, 66
Zona fasciculata of adrenal cortex, 25
Zona glomerulosa of adrenal cortex, aldosterone release from,
    25, 27, 34, 36
Zona reticularis of adrenal cortex, 25